LENS POWER IN ACTION

Robert A. Kraskin, O.D.

Reformatted and Edited
by
Paul A. Harris, O.D.
Gregory Kitchener, O.D.

Optometric Extension Program Foundation, Inc.

Copyright © 2003 Optometric Extension Program Foundation, Inc.

Printed in the United States

Published by the Optometric Extension Program
1921 E. Carnegie Ave., Suite 3-L
Santa Ana, CA 92705-5510

Managing editor: Sally Marshall Corngold
Cover design: Kathleen M. Patterson
Cover photo: Patrick D. Patterson

Library of Congress Cataloging-in-Publication Data
Kraskin, Robert A.
    Lens power in action / Robert A. Kraskin ; edited by Paul A. Harris, Gregory Kitchener.--Rev.ed.
      p. , cm.
    Includes bibliographical references.
    ISBN 0-943599-46-6
    1. Behavioral optometry. I. Harris, Paul, 1954 Jan 9- II. Kitchener, Gregory. III. Optometric Extension Program Foundation. IV. Title.
[DNLM: 1. Vision Disorders--rehabilitation. 2. Lenses. 3. Optometry--methods. WW140 K898L 2002]
RE960 .K736 2002
617.7'5--dc21
                                                                                      2002038138

Optometry is the health care profession specifically licensed by state law to prescribe lenses, optical devices and procedures to improve human vision. Optometry has advanced vision therapy as a unique treatment modality for the development and remediation of the visual process. Effective vision therapy requires extensive understanding of:

- the effects of lenses (including prisms, filters and occluders)
- the variety of responses to the changes produced by lenses
- the various physiological aspects of the visual process
- the pervasive nature of the visual process in human behavior

As a consequence, effective vision therapy requires the supervision, direction and active involvement of the optometrist.

Table of Contents

Preface · v

Introduction · vii

Chapter 1. The Uniqueness of Optometry · · · · · · · · · · · · · · 1

Chapter 2. The Analytical Value · · · · · · · · · · · · · · · · · 14

Chapter 3. What is a Visual Problem? · · · · · · · · · · · · · · · 24

Chapter 4. Preventive Optometric Care · · · · · · · · · · · · · · 34

Chapter 5. Stresspoint Retinoscopy · · · · · · · · · · · · · · · 39

Chapter 6. The Visual Process · · · · · · · · · · · · · · · · · 53

Chapter 7. Myopia: The Behavioral View · · · · · · · · · · · · · 60

Chapter 8. What Power Hath A Lens? · · · · · · · · · · · · · · · 73

Chapter 9. Yoked Prisms · · · · · · · · · · · · · · · · · · · 81

Chapter 10. The Behavioral Concept and Patient Management · · · 118

Chapter 11. Compensatory Lenses and Postural Alterations · · · · 142

Chapter 12. The Final Chapter: Only A Beginning · · · · · · · · · 161

PREFACE

"The fundamental hypothesis giving impetus to this series is that optometry is a unique profession. That which permits optometry to be a unique profession lies only within the appreciation and application of the behavioral vision care model."

These words written more than 20 years ago by Robert A. Kraskin, O.D., my father, can be found in the opening sentences of *Lens Power In Action*. More importantly, they capture his view of the power of the profession of optometry and its potential to shape human behavior. Many optometrists have benefited throughout the years from the concepts and principles outlined in this important series of papers. That so many of us have learned and matured as professional practitioners – and continue to learn and mature – by reading this series would be a source of great satisfaction to my father, if he was alive today.

My father practiced what he preached. *Lens Power In Action* exemplifies how he practiced optometry. In fact, the views expressed in this series were fundamental to his practice of optometry. As many of his colleagues know, he did not think of himself as a "behavioral" optometrist. He thought of himself, first and foremost, as "an" optometrist charged with the responsibility of ministering to his patients' visual needs. He embraced behavioral concepts as <u>an</u> optometrist and believed that all people could benefit from the clinical applications of the behavioral model outlined in *Lens Power In Action*.

As I learned from my father, the objective of scholarship, like that expressed in *Lens Power In Action*, is to stimulate new thinking. *Lens Power In Action* was written to raise <u>more</u> questions, not answer <u>all</u> questions. Typical of my father, however, he did not wait for others to raise questions about his thinking. Throughout *Lens Power In Action*, he asks the questions he thought his readers should raise. He believed that questions and discussion give birth to new ideas and new practical applications of theoretical concepts and principles. The practice to which he gave his heart and soul continues to operate like this today.

Lens Power In Action is not a sacred script to be put on a shelf and treated as a reverential icon. Rather, it is a working treatise destined to generate new thinking. The strength of the series is that it encourages all of us to reassess the behavioral vision care model and consider ways that we can better meet the needs of our patients, our colleagues, and our "unique" profession.

In many ways, *Lens Power In Action* is an unfinished work. Its basis is that we will continue to learn from our experiences of using lenses. By provoking more questions about the application of behavioral concepts, especially as they relate to lenses, *Lens Power In Action* will continue to expand our knowledge, our thinking, and the overall value of the profession of optometry.

That was the vision of my father: a profession that evolves with each new generation that is willing and committed to explore that which makes the profession of optometry so unique – the clinical application of the behavioral vision care model.

On behalf of the Kraskin family, I want to express our appreciation to the Optometric Extension Program (OEP) Foundation for publishing this series of papers again. We are proud that my father's thinking will be read and maybe even reread so that he can continue to provoke the type of questions that characterized his practice and continue to advance our profession. We also want to express our appreciation again to Thomas M. Smith, a family friend, who worked closely with my father to edit the original series of papers published in 1982.

Lens Power In Action demonstrates there is much work for all of us to do to expand the power of the behavioral vision care model. As my father often said, we must not fear spreading the word to others in our profession who may not know, appreciate, or understand the behavioral vision care model. But, we must also not be reluctant to reject compromise with our colleagues when such compromise jeopardizes the welfare of our patients who benefit most from the work we do and limit the scope of our profession.

Finally, the concepts outlined in *Lens Power In Action* are more than just my father's words. They also are his spirit. His life was committed to the exploration of new concepts and new applications of the behavioral vision care model. How we as another generation of optometrists grow our practices, mature as professionals, and enhance the clinical applications of the behavioral vision care model give new life to the spirit captured in *Lens Power In Action*. That would make him proud! And it continues to make his family, friends, and colleagues so proud of all he contributed to this very unique profession we call optometry.

Jeffrey Kraskin, O.D.

INTRODUCTION

The late Dr. Robert Kraskin originally wrote "Lens Power in Action" as 24 monthly chapters published over two years as part of the OEP *Curriculum II*. These chapters are referred to frequently and there have been numerous requests for reprints over the years. These requests were filled with loose-leaf photocopies. The decision to reissue these chapters in a book format to be made available to the profession developed from this ongoing interest.

There are many differences between preparing 24 chapters that are published separately and presenting the same material in a single volume. It would have been possible to simply reproduce the original work and ask the reader to bear with these differences. However, the editors felt that adapting the material to a book format would allow for a better presentation and flow of the material, with a broader appeal.

To accomplish this task, several chapters with related topics were consolidated. This occasionally meant changing the sequence of the original chapters and eliminating some of the transitions between chapters. Descriptive tags for individual probes of the Analytical Sequence were added. This was done for the benefit of readers who might be unfamiliar with the numbering system originated by Dr. Skeffington and used consistently by Dr. Kraskin.

Certain non-technical expressions and phrases were rewritten for clarity. The editors thought long and hard about these changes especially since it was not possible to consult with the original author. In each case the changes were felt to be consistent with Dr. Kraskin's expressed opinion and intent. No changes were made to any of the technical information, discussion, or data. Hopefully, on balance, the positive effects of any of the editorial changes will outweigh any potential negatives.

The editors would like to thank the Kraskin family for their help with many aspects of this task. We hope that this text does justice to Dr. Kraskin's contributions to the profession of optometry.

Paul A. Harris, O.D.
Gregory Kitchener, O.D.

CHAPTER 1
The Uniqueness of Optometry—Introduction

The fundamental hypothesis giving impetus to this text is that optometry is a unique profession. That which permits optometry to be a unique profession lies within the appreciation and application of the behavioral vision care model. This concept of vision recognizes that a critical element involved in the control and altering of behavior is a lens. There is no such thing as functioning within the framework of the behavioral concept or practicing a behavioral approach to optometry without an understanding of and utilization of lenses, including visual training. The appropriate utilization of lenses is absolutely essential to prevent visual problems and protect, control, maintain and enhance the visual process. The power of lenses to provide this level of benefits to people will be discussed, described and defined from a clinical vantage point, recognizing that the term "power" is used not in terms of dioptrics but in terms of value to the visual process. Thus, this book is entitled, *Lens Power in Action*.

A great contribution of the late Dr. A. M. Skeffington, former OEP Foundation Director of Education, was his unique ability to confound his colleagues and associates by raising the most provocative of questions. For example, it was Dr. Skeffington who asked us such questions as: What is vision? What is a visual problem? What is the value of binocularity? Such questioning led him to develop the search-model, which emerged subsequently as the behavioral concept in vision care.

What is the uniqueness of optometry? This is the most significant question posed by Dr. Skeffington, who long will be remembered as a great inquisitor and mind stimulator.

A profession exists and endures only if it provides a service and/or benefit that is unique and offered by no other profession. Optometry also, then, must offer a unique and valuable service if its status as a profession is to be maintained. Like all professions, optometry shares some of its tenets with other professions. However, optometry has a uniqueness of its own, that being the clinical application of the behavioral concept of vision. No other profession accurately claims such a function.

This book will echo the spirit of Dr. Skeffington by raising provocative and stimulating questions that could result in raised eyebrows, puzzled glances, and significant questions.

Already, your first question simply may be: "Why has the author decided to write about lenses?" Lenses? Yes, indeed! The author will write about lenses—lens power. Will this be a book, then, on optics, you ask? Is this a review course on prescribing glasses? When you consider all the other possible glamorous topics, like visual training, contact lenses, nutrition and even ocular pathology, why is the author concerning himself with something so mundane as lenses?

The notions of visual dysfunction and the prevention of visual problems emerge from the behavioral concept of vision. The behavioral concept of vision also recognizes that the visual process is developed and that it can be enhanced. That visual function and performance can be protected, controlled, and maintained is also a realization of the behavioral concept of vision. The clinical application of these notions is shared by no other concept or model of vision. Nor is it shared by any other profession.

Implied, then, is the recognition and understanding that the appropriate utilization of lenses is absolutely essential to prevent visual problems, and protect, control, maintain, and enhance the visual process. This book will address LENSES—that is, the optometrist's utilization of lenses for the purpose of providing people with benefits that exceed the more limited concepts of vision in which lenses are prescribed merely to compensate for an already existing condition.

To state it differently, yet more succinctly, the chapters will analyze comprehensively the "where, when and how" of lenses for purposes other than visual compensation. We shall deal with the influence of lenses on the behavior of people, with an emphasis on appreciating and understanding the dynamics involved. Hence, this volume is entitled *Lens Power in Action*. The emphasis will be clinical, including both the determination and application of lenses. The text also will consider theoretical and practical concepts of practice management.

As suggested earlier, this book will focus on questions—the basic questions of where, when, and how to determine and apply lenses. An attempt will be made to resolve the questions with pragmatic answers. Two questions you already may have asked are the following:

1. What is a lens? The use of the term lens or lenses in these chapters will refer, in general, to spheres, cylinders, and prisms. Specific identifica-

tion of the type of lenses discussed and considered will be indicated and identified.
2. What are compensatory lenses? It has been suggested already that the determination and application of compensatory lenses will not be a subject of these chapters. However, it is imperative that this term be appreciated. Compensatory lenses are lenses that, when prescribed, compensate for an existing, identifiable, and measurable "refractive" condition.

Unfortunately, corrective lenses, a term that is very misleading, has long been used instead of compensatory lenses, a more appropriate term. The assumption that lenses actually "correct" the condition is inappropriate and, in reality, could not be further from the truth. Optometrists interested in the behavioral aspects of vision care know that the term corrective is misused.

As an example, if a patient's unaided distance acuity is 20/200 and is restored to 20/20 with minus two diopter spheres, the patient may see clearly with the lenses, but the patient is still a myope. He was not "corrected;" he was "compensated." When compensatory lenses are utilized, the optometrist must avoid use of the false term corrective lenses. Perhaps, this term should be reserved for a more appropriate dynamic application when, utilizing some other means, the visual problem is truly "corrected." The optometrist should use the term refractive status, instead of refractive error, for the same reason. The optometrist does not "correct the refractive error;" instead he "compensates for the refractive status."

When reference is made to lens power, optometrists tend to think in terms of lens strength, diopters or prism diopters. The lens with greater power is one which has greater curvature or, in the case of a prism, a thicker base. The term "lens power" in this series has a different meaning. Fundamentally, lens power in action refers to the power of a lens to alter behavior. And, to the contrary, it is evident that small degrees of dioptrics, instead of strong lenses, are the rule, not the exception. The term power actually is used more synonymously with the word value. We are concerned with the value of any given lens as it relates to the behavior of a person. The greater the value to a person, the greater the power of the lens—but, again, not in terms of dioptrics. The power or value of a lens is derived from its ability to benefit a patient by preventing visual problems and protecting, controlling, maintaining, enhancing, and even remedying the visual system. Lens power is not the sum of its dioptrics.

Appreciating and utilizing the power of lenses is essential, but not only for the benefits afforded patients. It is also significant for the optometrist insofar as patient control, and patient and practice maintenance are concerned. First, the knowing optometrist is capable of offering and providing patients with benefits that are wanted and needed, but which were never previously provided because the patient never had access to the optometrist's knowledge of the behavioral concept.

Second, the knowing optometrist can determine when the benefits desired and needed by the patient are provided only by means of formalized visual training. This is extremely critical. Not all optometrists offer formalized visual training as a service in their offices. The need and responsibility for intraprofessional referral certainly has been encouraged and emphasized.

This increased emphasis has prevailed for at least two major reasons. First, some optometrists are reluctant to refer their patients to another colleague although they are unable to provide the essential level of care that might solve the patients' problems; and, second, some optometrists do not recognize that a patient has a visual problem that could be solved if referred to a colleague who provides visual training.

As, first, optometric reluctance to refer was reduced, and, second, optometrists' awareness of patient benefits to be derived as a product of referral for visual training was increased, the number of optometric intraprofessional referrals increased. However, this created a new consequence that, on the surface, may seem shocking to some, and that is the problem of over-referral for visual training. An over-referral would be the case of a patient with needs that the optometrist can service by utilizing means other than the more complex and involved approach of formalized visual training—in other words, a patient whose problems can be solved by the POWER OF LENSES.

The *behavioral concept* of vision tells us that visual training can enhance the function of vision and improve the visual performance of every human being. Practically, however, everyone does not have needs that require visual training. If all the patients who wanted visual training were accepted for visual training, regardless of their need, there would not be enough optometrists to service them. Nor would there be sufficient time and space in the offices that provide visual training to care for those who truly have needs that can be satisfied only by visual training.

To be accepted as a patient for visual training, the patient, first, must have a need or needs that can be satisfied only by visual training; and, second, and most important, the patient and/or parents (in the case of a child) must be aware of this need and desire the benefits that are the products of visual training. The optometrist can be sure of satisfied, excited and enthusiastic patients if these simple guidelines are followed.

On the basis of a normal population distribution of a general optometric practice, realistically only about 20% have needs that can be satisfied only by visual training. These are patients for whom the benefits to be gained are well worth the effort, time and money required for formalized visual training. Incidentally, contrary to popular opinion, these patients are primarily adults and young adults, not children.

However, intraprofessional referral should not be discouraged, and it is hoped that, as a result of this book, the optometrist will encourage referrals from his colleagues and also refer to his colleagues for visual training if he does not already provide this service within his established practice. Additionally, it is hoped that the reader will broaden his base of knowledge so that he can determine more adequately when the power of lenses alone will satisfy patient needs and when formalized visual training is required and, in this way, avoid over-referral.

Recognizing, of course, that he cannot solve the patient's problems, the referring optometrist, on the other hand, should not refer the patient specifically for visual training. Instead, he should refer the patient for consultation, just in case the patient's problems can be solved by utilizing the *power of lenses*. This will avoid embarrassment, as well as the need to accept a referred patient for visual training when his problems can be satisfied by utilizing a more simple approach. These recommendations are the product of experience and true appreciation of the behavioral concept and the power of lenses. If allowed, they will lead to superb intraprofessional relations and very enthusiastic patients.

It was noted that optometry could stand alone as an independent profession if it maintains its uniqueness by providing a service and/or benefit offered by no other profession.

Actually, optometry has dual roles. Not only is optometry a profession; it is also the discipline of vision.

As a profession, optometry, by definition, specializes in the examination, diagnosis and treatment of conditions of the visual system. Most, if not all, optometrists can accept this definition which was formulated by the American Optometric Association (AOA). However, optometry's uniqueness is not inherent in the definition; nor can it be assumed. The interpretation and significance of this definition is derived from the point of view or concept of vision of any given optometrist.

Earlier it was suggested that the uniqueness of optometry and the justification and rationalization for the preservation of optometry as an independent profession depends on the optometrist's clinical application of the behavioral concept of vision. It was suggested that optometry is unique because of the optometrist's appreciation and application of lenses, the product of the optometrist's understanding and utilization of the behavioral concept. In other words, the optometrist understands and applies the power of lenses to provide benefits to patients, either by lenses alone or lenses as an element of formalized visual training. (Hopefully, it is already appreciated that there is no such thing as visual training without the utilization of lenses.)

References have been made to such terms as (1) the behavioral optometrist, (2) behavioral optometry, and (3) the behavioral concept. Of course, this implies (and correctly so) that there are concepts and approaches to optometry other than the behavioral. Sometimes referred to as the *dynamic functional concept of vision*, the behavioral concept has emerged over the years as a product of empirical clinical activity and inquisitive minds. The late Dr. A. M. Skeffington spearheaded this movement.

Earlier concepts of vision, (1) the optical concept and (2) the accommodative- convergence concepts, were based on assumptions rather than the "knowns" from which clinical directives were derived. As years passed, many became aware of the limitations, restrictions and contradictions imposed on patients by the applications of these earlier notions of vision. Behavior did not conform to conventional wisdom; questions arose; and, recognizing the inconsistencies between theory and reality, inquisitive professionals searching for solutions sought to untangle the imposed web.

This will not be a treatise on historical review and development of optometry as this is simply not the purpose, nor the intent, of this text. But, it is important to note that the behavioral concept emerged as a product of a search model. It was not created first by any one individual and then followed by attempts to fit people to the model. And, finally, it should be noted that the concept is neither complete, final, nor capable of answering all questions that arise as a product of observing behavior. It is a model that explains and guides the clinical activities of the optometrist.

A behavioral approach to optometry, by definition, is the optometric clinical application of the dynamic functional concept of vision, the Skeffington approach.

To facilitate a review for the optometrist familiar with the behavioral concept and to provide an initial insight for the neophyte, the following are the fundamental tenets of the dynamic functional concept of vision.

1. The visual process is dominant
2. Vision is developed
3. Vision is motor
4. Vision is an emergent
5. Visual problems are products of interference or inadequacy in development and/or interference in that which has been developed and, thus visual problems are representations of adaptations.
6. Ophthalmic lenses may be used for:
   a. Prevention
   b. Protection, control and maintenance
   c. Remediation
   d. Enhancement
   e. Compensation
7. The process of vision is trainable and this process may be mediated by means of:
   a. Developmental guidance
   b. Utilization of lenses
   c. Formalized visual training

One additional definition is essential before continuing. As stated earlier, optometry is the discipline of vision. But, what is vision? The definition is as broad and as meaningful as the concept from which the term is derived. The term itself has meanings other than those related to the vision-care professions.

The word "vision" is equated by some with visual acuity, especially if the concept of vision is other than the behavioral. This author has overheard even optometrists periodically discuss a patient and say that the patient has "20/20 vision," although they really meant that the patient's "visual acuity" was 20/20.

In the listing of the foregoing tenets of the dynamic functional concept of vision, numbers 2, 3, 4, and 7 refer specifically to vision as defined. These tenets state: vision is developed; vision is motor; vision is an emergent; and vision is trainable. Any definition of vision must incorporate these basic tenets in order to be consistent with the behavioral concept.

The author defines VISION as follows: the deriving of meaning and the directing of action as a product of the processing of information triggered by a selected band of radiant energy.

Lens power in action is best evidenced and discussed by using actual patients' records and case studies. The following is an excellent example for beginning this course.

Vicki D, age 17, was referred by an optometrist in her hometown (nearly 100 miles from this author's office) for consultation and possibly for visual training. She reported an awareness of periodic vertical diplopia. Recently, Vicki's friends told her that her eyes did not always point in the same direction. As a child, Vicki's parents noted periodic vertical deviation of her eyes. Until the recent optometric examination by the referral source however, she never had any vision care or examination. She experienced frontal headaches during the last two years which occurred when she was tired and under visual demands such as schoolwork. Her eyes itched and burned and she had pain in her upper back and neck when she tired. Often she experienced general fatigue without good cause.

Although Vicki can see clearly, she is aware of a delay in "focus" when her vision shifts from near to far. Reading makes her sleepy and she avoids it if possible. She is a slow reader and she must reread for meaning. Vicki, a senior in high school, gets good grades but she must work very hard to attain these grades.

External and ophthalmoscopic examination revealed no evidence of pathology.

Unaided visual acuity: at far, right, left and both eyes 20/20; at near, right 20/30, left 20/20, both eyes 20/30.

Convergence nearpoint: 4 feet, right eye deviating; diplopia reported.

Cover test: at far, orthophoria; at near, vertical deviancy, tending to fixate with right eye with left hypotropia; can alternate to fixate with left eye with right hypertropia.

Ocular motility: full eye movement, either eye, but jerky and uneven.

#3 (habitual distance phoria)--2 exo

#4 (distance retinoscopy)	OD +0.25 -0.25 x 180 OS +0.25 -0.50 x 180
#5 (retinoscopy at 20 inches)	OD +1.50 -0.25 x 180 OS +1.75 -0.50 x 180 (diplopia)
#7 (distance subjective)	OD +0.75 -0.25 x 10 OS +0.25

#8 (distance phoria through #7)--1 exo

#9, #10, #11 (distance base out and base in prism ranges)--diplopia; single with 2 prism diopters base-up

#12 (distance vertical phoria)--unstable; 2 right hyperphoria

#13A (near habitual phoria) and #13B (near phoria through #7)--suppression

#14A (unfused cross cylinder)   OD +0.50 -0.25 x 10
                                OS +1.00

#16 and #17 (near base-out and base-in prism ranges)--left suppression

#18 (near vertical phoria)--3 right hyperphoria

Upon general observation, the following asymmetric posturing was noted: head tilted forward and to the left; it was easier for her to tilt her head to the left than to the right. When she tilts her head to the right, she reports blur; with her head in a straight position, diplopia is reported, but vision becomes single when her head is permitted to return to habitual position.

She has single vision on the Motor Fields test with eyes to the right; vertical diplopia increases in separation as she turns her eyes to the left. The Stereo Fly is flat, and she has no response on the Wirt stereo test.

The raw data has been presented. How would you interpret and analyze this data? What is your diagnosis? What are your recommendations?

Take a moment to think about how you would approach caring for Vicki D.

With one exception, the raw data gathered at the time of Vicki D's examination are presented. Before revealing the author's interpretation, analysis, diagnosis and recommendations, it should be realized that appropriate recommendations were made and implemented. The patient returned three months later for a scheduled, programmed, progress case study which revealed the following:

She no longer has headaches or any other form of discomfort. Close work is easier and she gets her schoolwork done faster. She experiences less sleepiness with reading and, in fact, it takes her longer to tire. She is aware of a significant increase in her efficiency and she is not aware of diplopia at any time.

Unaided visual acuity:

At far: Right, left and both eyes 20/20

At near: Right, left and both eyes 20/20

Convergence nearpoint: 6 inches, right eye deviating; diplopia reported; recovery at 8 inches

Cover test: Ortho at far and near

Far:

#3 (habitual distance phoria)--1 eso   #13A--2 exo

#4 (retinoscopy)   OD +0.25 sph.
                            OS +0.25 -0.50 x 180

#5 (retinoscopy at 20 inches)   OD +2.00 sph.
                                OS +2.00 -0.50 x 180

#7 (subjective)   OD +0.50 sph.
                            OS +0.50 -0.25 x 180

#8 (phoria through #7)--Orthophoria

#9 (base-out blur)--20

#10 (base-out break/recovery)--29/1

#11 (base-in break/recovery)--7/2

#12 (vertical phoria)--½ right hyperphoria

Near:

#13B (phoria through #7)--5 exo

#16A (base-out blur)--X   #16B (base-out break/recovery)--18/2

#17B (base-in break/recovery)--19/6

#18 (vertical phoria)--2 right hyperphoria

Wirt Stereo Test
   With Plano OU: #8
   With #7 OU: #9

If a comparison is made between the information and data collected at the original examination and this progress case study, it should be obvious that the differences in performance and function are rather dramatic. In fact, the differences are remarkable.

But, how was the data initially interpreted, analyzed, and diagnosed? And what was recommended and done for Vicki D? This will be revealed in reverse order. First, it will be revealed what was recommended and done and then we will investigate the "Why."

Vicki D was returned to the referring optometrist at the conclusion of the initial examination following analysis and diagnosis with a prescription for lenses and the recommendation that the lenses be used for all near-centered visual activities. The prescription was: OU +0.62 spheres.

Knowing now what was prescribed and recommended, certain questions must, of necessity, arise:

1. How was such a prescription determined?
2. Were the changes that took place expected?
3. How was the patient viewed optometrically?
   And how was the data analyzed and interpreted?

It was stated earlier that all of the raw data gathered at the time of the initial examination were presented with one exception. As it turns out, this was a very important piece of information. More specifically, this one exception represented the stresspoint retinoscopic observation. The stresspoint retinoscopy (SPR) measurement was OU +0.62 sphere.

The reader may or may not be familiar with SPR, its technique and its significance. The specific procedure will be discussed and described in a later chapter. It is important to appreciate for now that SPR is one of a number of procedures used to determine the counter-stress (or stress-relieving) lens prescription. Depending on the needs of the person and the status of his visual behavior, SPR may be considered for prevention, protection, remediation or enhancement purposes. Due to a personal bias, the author contends that SPR is the most direct means of determining this information. It is the primary and, usually, only means used by this author to determine lens value.

Although such a dioptric value as OU +0.62 spheres was determined by SPR, how was its value rationalized? And, was it really predictable that such benefits would result as a product of its use? The value and importance attributed to the utilization of "low plus" lenses has been associated for years with the work and teachings of the Optometric Extension Program (OEP). In fact, some think that OEP and the use of plus lenses are equivalent. Yet, nothing could be further from the truth.

On the other hand, as a product of pragmatic investigation and utilization, the opportunities afforded by the OEP have revealed the significance of lenses on behavior—hence, this whole series on the *power of lenses*. This case study certainly is an excellent example of lens power in action. But why?

Let us finally view this data optometrically by examining the author's analysis and interpretation as well as conclusions. A number of unusual facets were associated with this patient's data, i.e., (1) reason for initial referral, (2) vertical diplopia and early history of vertical deviancy, and (3) lack of typical binocular data usually derived from standard probes of the analytical examination and available for interpretation. Despite this, the available data were capable of adequate interpretation on the basis of a solid behavioral concept and a personal conviction as to its validity and reliability because behavior is highly predictable.

Considering the early history and evaluation of extraocular muscle activity in association with observed postures, the conclusion was drawn that there are neuro-motor deficits resulting in either an overactive or underactive musculature that was probably congenital and to which the patient had made prior postural adaptation. However, the symptoms of discomfort, fatigue, relative inefficiency, more recent observation of diplopia, and peer observation of vertically deviating eyes suggested the possibility that present visual behavior was relatively non-embedded. If so, then the present visual behavior would be highly amenable to appropriate counter-stress lenses. Although it was impossible to appraise the data as usually done to determine the degree of embeddedness, certain bits and pieces were rationalized and put together, which led to this assumption.

Present discomfort symptoms for two years suggested relative non-embeddedness. Recent peer observation of vertical deviancy and personal awareness of diplopia also suggested this. The type of performance observed and noted in the process of an analytical examination also suggested this. If postural adaptation in earlier years was embedded, chances were great that binocular data behind the phoropter would have been available, just as data were available following the use of the recommended lenses.

Additionally, some comments should be made relative to the discomfort factors. It has been said (S. Howard Bartley) that visual discomfort arises when visual efficiency is lower than that satisfactory to the individual.[1] Another way of phrasing the same description is that visual discomfort exists when the level of demand is greater than the freedom to meet the demand. Recognizing that the more non-embedded the behavior the less efficient the behavior, it then can be suggested that the level of demand within the last couple of years increased and created a non-embedded behavior which resulted in an upset of prior adaptation and a manifestation of the behavior as revealed by the examination. The author summarized his personal notes and observations, made recommendations, and what follows is taken directly from the original write-up of the data.

The optometric evaluation of the collected data and information reveals the evidence of initial physical impairment and limitation of extraocular muscle activity, probably congenital, to which Vicki D has made postural adaptation. The discomfort symptoms probably are not related to this earlier existing congenital condition, but are the result of a stress-induced vision disability resulting in limitation in information processing, the discomfort arising as an alarm signal because the level of demand has been greater than the freedom to meet the demand.

Recommendations: Prescribe appropriate counter-stress lenses in single vision form to be used initially for remedial purposes; the use of such lenses for ALL NEAR-CENTERED VISUAL DEMANDS will reduce current stress, providing increase in comfort, increased sustaining ability on near tasks, probable increased efficiency, and probable restoration of prior postural adaptation, alleviating diplopia and vertical shifting of eyes. In addition, use of such lenses will provide control and protection against additional adverse adaptation. Return in three months for reevaluation examination and determination of any additional needs, if any, related to vision care.

In the next chapter we shall continue to explore the power of lenses and begin to gain insight into "what does a lens do." We shall continue to use patient data as a vehicle. In addition, we shall investigate in more detail the information that is available to us from the complete optometric examination so as to better understand human behavior, and, more specifically, the visual behavior of people.

Reference
1. Bartley SH. Principles of Perception. 2nd Ed. Harper & Row, 1969:457-458.

CHAPTER 2
The Analytical Value

Brett B, age 9 years, 2 months, was seen for his initial, complete optometric examination by this author in September at the beginning of his third grade in school. He was examined two months earlier by a non-optometric examiner. Although his parents suspected visual problems, the non-optometric examiner made no diagnosis or recommendations and, instead, pronounced him to be "fit-as-a-fiddle," with 20/20 distance visual acuity, healthy eyes and no ocular defects.

Case History

The case history reveals the following information about Brett: sees clearly and has no symptoms of discomfort; has always attended private schools; repeated first grade due (supposedly) to age and maturation level; although doing fairly well in school, it was reported that reading development was slow and performance was lower than his peers; tutored some for reading in the past school year; observed recently getting very close to desk work and holding books very close to his face; loses place when reading and uses his finger as a marker.

The investigation of eye health status revealed the eyes and adnexa to be free from pathology and abnormality.

Case Findings

The data gathered from the optometric examination follows:

Unaided visual acuity at far and near: 20/20 right, left and both eyes

Cover test: ortho far and near

Convergence nearpoint: 3 inches, both eyes deviating out and diplopia reported; recovery at 6 inches

Ocular motility: pursuit movements were full and unrestricted but very poor; fixations were very poor, continually overshooting

Visual Abilities (Telebinocular, DB series)
    DB10 (pig and dog): both present
    DB8 (line and ball): suppression; no hyperphoria
    DB6D (stereopsis): #12
    BU21: (stereo/suppression test) patient suppressed
    DB3 and DB2 (signboards): 20/17
    DB9 (far) (arrow and numbers): unstable at #7
    DB9 (near) (arrow and numbers): unstable at #2

DB 5K (3 balls at near): 4 balls in eso

Wirt stereo: #7

The Analytical Examination

#3 (distance habitual phoria)--3 eso   #13A (near habitual phoria)--2 eso

#4 (retinoscopy)--OU +0.25 sph.

#5 (retinoscopy at 20 inches)--OU +1.75 sph.

#7 (subjective)--OU +0.50 sph.

#8 (phoria through #7)--1 eso
  (Control at far: OU Plano)

#9 (base out blur)--11

#10 (base-out break/recovery)--21/6

#11 (base-in break/recovery)--2/-2

#13B (near phoria through #7)--Ortho

#14A (unfused cross cylinder)   OD +1.50
                                 OS +1.75

#15A (phoria through 14A)--5 exo

#14B (fused cross cylinder)   OD +1.25
                                OS +1.50

#15B (phoria through 14B)--7 exo

 (Control at near: OU Plano)

#16A (base-out blur) X   #16B (base-out break/recovery) 22/3

#17A (base-in blur) X   #17B (base-in break/recovery) 12/3

#20 (minus lens to blur out)-- -2.00

#21 (plus lens to blur out)-- +2.75

Stresspoint Retinoscopy
  OU +0.75 provided best balance

Book Retinoscopy
  3rd reader level was effortful with .50D against motion

The data from Brett's initial optometric examination has been presented. Now, let us pause, reflect and raise some questions. Does Brett have a visual problem? What are his needs? Will an optometric program of care satisfy his needs? If so, what optometric program of care is appropriate? The data presented is complete insofar as Brett's examination is concerned. This is not to imply that this example is representative of every patient's examination in the author's office. Of course, diagnostic study data depends on age, patient history and the adequacy of information gathered routinely. As long as a patient in Brett's age range is capable of binocular investigation, the examination represents the minimum. Additionally, the minimum is more the rule rather than the exception. The author's attitude regarding an optometric examination always is to get the maximum information in the minimum amount of time. Assuming binocular capability, the following is representative of an outline of the optometric diagnostic examination:

1. Eye health investigation
2. Visual performance tests, including visual acuity, cover tests, convergence nearpoint break and recovery and ocular pursuits and fixations
3. Visual abilities (Telebinocular and Wirt stereo test)
4. The analytical examination (OEP 21-point)
5. Stresspoint retinoscope

The above is modified as required by such factors as age and need. The ultimate purpose of the optometric examination from the behavioral point of view is as follows: to appraise adequacy of vision development; to evaluate the adequacy of the visual process to perform; to gain insight into the status of visual behavior; and to understand the person's mode of adaptation. This is the sum of an optometric diagnosis resulting from the optometrist's evaluation of the gathered data. That which is done in the course of an optometric examination is determined primarily by the concept of vision from which the optometrist is operating. The concept guides the examiner and influences what he does, what he looks for, and what is recommended for treating the patient.

Therefore, the gathered data may seem to some readers incomplete and inadequate. This may create some degree of frustration and it may lead to a wish that the author had done additional specific performance testing in order to draw conclusions and make recommendations. And yet, to others, the examination may seem overly complete and they may wonder why the author wasted so much time and energy.

Let us now return to the questions posed earlier and answer them from the behavioral optometrist's point of view. This will provide an insight and understanding of the answers.

1. Does Brett have a visual problem?
   Answer: Yes

2. What are his needs?
   Answers:
   a. To function more efficiently in reading
   b. To avoid losing his place when reading
   c. To eliminate the need to use a finger as a marker
   d. To be in better postural balance in near-centered tasks
   e. To prevent additional adverse adaptation
3. Will an optometric program of care satisfy his needs?
   Answer: Yes
4. If so, what optometric program of care is appropriate
   Answer: LENSES

To understand Brett's visual behavior and his visual problem, and to ultimately satisfy his needs with appropriate optometric care, attention must be directed to a brief consideration of the etiology of conditions of the vision system.

In Chapter 1, the fundamental tenets of the behavioral concept were listed. Tenet #5 stated that visual problems are products of interference or inadequacy in development and/or interference in that which has been developed. More specifically, this tenet differentiates two categories of dysfunction, which, as a product of differential diagnosis based upon data and information gleaned from the optometric examination, can be revealed. Thus, for etiological purposes, we differentiate (1) vision development problems from (2) stress-induced visual problems. And, differentiation is critical insofar as understanding, recommending and applying appropriate optometric care. (A later chapter will deal more specifically with the consideration of vision development problems.)

It can be said, then, that it appears that a rather small percentage of visual dysfunctions is related to thwarting the developmental process of vision, whereas the vast majority of vision disabilities are the products of adverse response to stress. The prime stressor agent appears to be the biologically unacceptable visually near-centered task. Years ago, this type of visual dysfunction was referred to as a nearpoint visual problem.

When one is vulnerable (and vulnerability is a product of development), one may respond physiologically to stress imposed by the stressor agent and, as a result, adversely adapt. D. B. Harmon phrased this process as "growing along a line of stress to reduce stress." There are two primary "avenues" of adaptation to stress imposed by the visually near-centered task. The first is myopia and the other is the syndrome of reduced visual efficiency. The latter is the most common. Both of these will be discussed in later chapters. It is most important for now to appreciate that the process of adaptation is a function of time.

The Analytical Value

The earliest stage of adverse response is referred to as being non-embedded (i.e., not habituated) and, in due course of time as adaptation takes place, the behavior becomes more embedded (i.e., habituated). The more non-embedded the behavior the easier it is with simple means to alter and/or rectify the behavior. The more embedded, the less amenable and less easy it is to alter behavior with simple means. Another way of specifically stating the realities of it all from an optometric viewpoint is that the more non-embedded the behavior the more the value of lenses; the more embedded, the less the value of lenses alone and the more the need for formalized visual training.

With the foregoing serving as a minimal review for some and a minimal introduction for others, we shall turn our attention to the analytical examination as we gradually analyze and understand Brett's data and then provide an optometric program of care for him.

The analytical examination sequence for this author is considered as only one "test" comprised of numerous investigatory probes (namely #3 through #21). The behavioral optometrist always conducts the analytical examination sequence completely, and never in part, as long as the patient is capable of responding to all the probes. And, most significantly (since it is a psychometric sequence), it must be done always as it has been described both as to instructional sets and physical set-up. Only then is it truly significant in permitting the appraisal of visual behavior.

Appropriate analysis of the data available from the analytical examination sequence provides direct insight as to (1) whether or not a stress-induced dysfunction exists and (2) the degree of embeddedness. The author knows of no better direct means from which the same information and insight can be derived and determined. For more specific and elaborate information relative to the interpretation of this data, the reader is referred to the 1980 Revised Edition of *The Behavioral Optometry Approach to Lens Prescribing* by Homer Hendrickson, O.D., (revised and reprinted in 1996 as *A Field Manual in Clinical Optometry: Guidelines for Clinical Testing, Lens Prescribing and Vision Care* by Earl P. Schmitt, M.A., O.D., Ed.D., D.O.S., which is available from the OEP Foundation).

Analyzing Brett's examination data, it was concluded that he showed signs of a stress-induced visual problem that was non-embedded. The non-embedded syndrome suggested that the disability is of relative recent origin and that it was probably created during the latter part of the former school year. The dysfunction is representative of restriction in information processing. The end result is reduced visual efficiency. There was no evidence suggesting a more deep-seated vision development problem, and it is highly probable that earlier delays in learning were related to maturation rather than dysfunction or inadequacy in vision development. If the diagnosis and data interpretation is correct, the correct use of appropriate lenses should be extremely significant since behavior is highly predictable and his visual behavior is so non-embedded.

On the other hand, if Brett had been viewed from a more conventional concept of vision, the chances are great that such an examiner would not detect, diagnose or even appreciate the evidence of an existing visual problem. Brett's behavior would never have been related to visual dysfunction. If the reader recalls, this was, in fact, the case. His examination two months earlier resulted in no diagnosis and no recommendations. It was reported that he had 20/20 distance visual acuity, healthy eyes and no ocular defects.

The author's summation and recommendations taken directly from the case write-up were as follows:

The optometric evaluation of the collected data and information reveals the non-embedded syndrome of the stress-induced visual problem associated with reduced and restricted visual efficiency as a product of interference in information processing. Recommendation: provide appropriate counter-stress lenses in dual focus form to be used initially during all indoor activity for therapeutic purposes. The use of such lenses will reduce current stress, permitting and providing improvement in visual function as well as reversal of present impairment. Anticipate increased and improved visual efficiency. Continued utilization of appropriate counter-stress lenses will ultimately provide control and protection (preventive approach) against additional stress induced by the visually near-centered demands. Return for reevaluation examination (progress case study) in three months.

From the above recommendations, it can be seen that the need was to prescribe lenses in bifocal form so that (1) the lenses would be on his face constantly during the time he was most likely to be doing near-centered activity, and (2) being in bifocal form, he could not have the opportunity to misuse the glasses as he would if they were in single vision form.

Initially, these lenses are being used for therapeutic purposes (remedial and enhancement) and must be used for all near-centered demands if benefits are to be gained. When the visual problem is alleviated, appropriate counter-stress lenses (possibly the same prescription) will be used for preventive purposes. Straight-top 35 mm bifocals with segment height at the lower edge of the pupils were prescribed. The prescription was: OU Plano, add +0.75 D.

In summation, this case demonstrates that the prescription for lenses used as a counter-stress agent was determined by means of the stresspoint retinoscope test. The value of such lenses is determined by the analysis of the data derived from the analytical examination sequence.

The value of the behavioral use of lenses is highly predictable and that it is based on insight and the analysis of data accumulated from the analytical examination sequence. The less embedded the case, the greater the expectations from the use of lenses; the more embedded, the converse is true.

However, contrary to some beliefs and misconceptions, the actual dioptric power of any lens prescription utilized from the behavioral point of view is nowhere to be found within the findings of the analytical examination sequence. Frequently, the lens prescription is determined by professional judgment from insights gained by observing performance; sometimes this method has been referred to as feeling tone. Others seek more specific and direct clinical means of determining this prescription. Such examples are as follows: Macdonald Form Field Card, MEM retinoscopy, Bell retinoscopy, and stresspoint retinoscopy. (Stresspoint retinoscopy will be considered in detail in a forthcoming chapter.)

However, these methods are limited to providing information relative to the spherical lens values, usually plus powers, and referred to as the counter-stress or stress-relieving lenses. None of these methods provide insight to additional elements frequently included within the prescription of therapeutic purposes, such as prism values. This aspect will be considered in a later chapter.

It has been claimed and taught, erroneously, that such lens prescriptions are to be found within the findings of the analytical examination sequence and that they would be equivalent to the lenses prescribed based on the "Skeffington Analytical Sequence (SAS)," which involves "checking, chaining and typing" and applying the seven directives for successful lens fitting. Yet, nothing could be further from the truth or reality.

When utilized for the purpose as stated (i.e., successful lens fitting), the Skeffington Analytical Sequence is as valuable today as it was when it was first formulated. Successful lens fitting means determining and providing a pair of lenses that satisfy minimal levels of need and can be worn comfortably without complaint by the patient. It is still, to this day, the most efficient and effective optometric method to determine and provide the level of vision care required for which it was designed. But, it was not designed as a means to evaluate visual performance and to determine lens values from the behavioral concept. In fact, the SAS was derived from an accommodative-convergence concept in the late 1920's and early 1930's. This method is far superior to any other, such as graphical, accommodative convergence to accommodation ratio (AC/A), or even "flying by the seat of the pants" method and the "7 and 4, out the door" method, if the only level of care desired on the part of the clinician for his patients is the "minimal." Yet, it should be appreciated that the same analytical procedures are absolutely necessary to approach the patient from the behavioral point of view. The methods and data are the same; however, the ordering and interpretation of the data are different.

Case Study: Brett

Brett's initial case study data shows that the SAS method would have classified him as a B2 case typing. This means that #11 and #17B are low and the directive is to cut plus at far and give full plus at near. Analysis of the data and application of the other directives would dictate that no lens power be provided at far and that the maximum available plus at near is +0.37D. Prescribing this amount of lens power, at least, would have been better and actually more productive to Brett than doing nothing. But, "doing nothing" was the recommendation from a more conventional point of view. You will recall that it was the non-optometric examiner who made no diagnosis and no recommendations, who found 20/20 acuity, healthy eyes, no ocular defects; who DID NOTHING.

Recall that the behavioral point of view provided Brett with dual focus lenses to be used constantly when indoors. The prescription was OU Plano, add +0.75, straight top 35 mm (ST-35) bifocals with segment height even with lower edge of pupils. He was programmed to be seen for a progress case study three months later.

Brett's next office visit was delayed due to the winter vacation period until the end of the first semester of the current school year. The appointment was scheduled in early February, and the following was reported and revealed:

A. Patient and Parent Interview

Lenses have been worn as instructed. He sees clearly and reports no discomfort. He is doing very well in school and he no longer loses his place when reading, nor does he use his finger as a marker. No problem is noted in postural approach to near-centered tasks.

B. Visual Performance

Unaided visual acuity at far and near: 20/20 right, left and both eyes

Convergence nearpoint: 1 inch, both eyes deviating out and diplopia reported; recovery at 3 inches

Ocular motility: pursuit movement and fixations were excellent

Telebinocular: no evidence of suppressions

    DB4K 3 balls
    DB5K (with Rx) 3 balls

Wirt StereoTest
    With Plano OU: #8
    With Rx OU: #9

C. The Analytical Examination

#3 (distance habitual phoria)--1 eso   #13A (Plano) (near habitual phoria)--6 eso

#4 (retinoscopy)--OU +0.25 spheres

#5 (retinoscopy at 20 inches)--OU +1.50 spheres

#7 (subjective)--OU +0.50 spheres
   (Control at far, OU Plano)

#8 (phoria through #7)--½ eso

#9 (base-out blur)--X

#10 (base-out break/recovery)--17/6

#11 (base-in break/recovery)--4/0

#13B (near phoria with Rx)--½ exo

#14A (unfused cross cylinder)--OU +2.25

#15A (phoria through #14A)--8 exo

#14B (fused cross cylinder)--OU +2.00

#15B (phoria through #14B)--8 exo
   (Control at near, OU +0.75)

#16A (base-out blur)--X   #16B (base out break/recovery) 21/7

#17A (base-in blur)--X   #17B (base in break/recovery) 15/8

#20 (minus lens to blur out) (from Plano)-- -3.00

D. Stresspoint Retinoscopy

OU +0.75 provided best balance

It will be noted that the data reported above in C, gathered during the Progress Case Study (PCS) is not a complete analytical sequence (#19 and #21 were omitted).

Following is an explanation and rationale for these omissions.

The data of the analytical examination serves two primary purposes: (1) From the data of the complete analytical and with the application of the seven directives of lens application, a "safe" lens can be determined which is equivalent to our alternative No. 1, the conventional approach. (2) The behavioral interpretation of the collected data permits one to know the status of visual behavior of the patient.

At the time of the PCS, only those parts of the analytical required by the examiner for comparison so related to the visual behavior are repeated, and a complete analytical, considering time consumed and value gained, is not a necessity. The purpose of the PCS is to identify change in status, and has nothing to do with the determination of a "safe" lens.

The patient and parents were pleased with this program of optometric care. The predicted benefits were being evidenced. Because of the period of time permitted for the use of these therapeutic lenses, the author, however, was somewhat disappointed in the analytical findings in spite of the fact that significant changes occurred. Additional questions revealed that the lenses possibly were not being used for ALL INDOOR activity as required. It was suggested that the lenses were used less indoors at home than at school. Therefore, Brett was instructed to continue his therapeutic program and use his lenses more conscientiously for all indoor activities. No change in lenses was required. Although he is still in the process of physiological improvement, he is not free from impairment. This is to be expected in time as a product of continued utilization of these lenses. He was programmed to be seen once again at the beginning of the next school year for a reevaluation examination in seven months.

Obviously, then, the parents were instructed to call if any questionable behavior or performance were noted prior to the next examination. If at that time the visual behavior is seen as being stable and free from impairment, he will continue to use appropriate counter-stress lenses for preventive purposes for all near-centered demands. The data from the examination will determine whether the preventive lenses will be different from the current therapeutic lenses. He will be seen next in one year if he is free from impairment.

CHAPTER 3
What Is A Visual Problem?

The following case study sets the stage for our discussion of what a visual problem is. Susan D, age 18 years, 3 months, was seen for a complete optometric examination during her winter break from college. She is a freshman in college and has never had any form of vision and/or eye examination. The case history was reported as follows: she sees clearly at far and near, and she is not aware of any delay in clearing when shifting from near to far or far to near. Generally, she has no headaches but she has been aware of tired and itching eyes since she entered college. She was a "B" student in high school but has had great difficulty in coping with college-level demands. Her first semester in college (just completed) was very poor. She has always been a slow reader and she is aware of having to reread for meaning. She has great difficulty in concentrating. Susan reports that she always learns easiest by listening and discussing rather than reading and studying.

The investigation of eye health status revealed that the eyes and adnexa were free from pathology and abnormality.

The data gathered from the optometric examination follows.

Unaided visual acuity at far: right and left poor 20/20, both eyes 20/20

Unaided visual acuity at near: 20/20 right, left and both eyes.

Cover Test: ortho far and near

Convergence nearpoint: 2 inches, left eye deviates and reports diplopia, recovery at 4 inches.

Ocular motility: pursuit movements were full, spastic and jerky; fixations were poor and erratic

Visual abilities (Telebinocular, DB series)

    DB 10 (pig and dog): suppression
    DB 8 (line and ball): suppression
    DB 4K (3 balls): reports 3 balls with suppression
    DB 6D (stereopsis): #12
    DB 3D (signboard): 20/25, improved to 20/22 with left eye occluded
    DB 2D (signboard): 20/20, improved to 20/17 with right eye occluded
    BU 21: suppression

DB9 (far arrow and numbers): #9 stable
DB9 (near arrow and numbers): #4 stable
DB 5K (3 balls near): 3 balls with suppression

Wirt stereo #9

The Analytical Examination

#3 (habitual distance phoria)--2 exo (habitual near phoria) #13A--1 exo

#4 (distance retinoscopy) OD +0.25 sph.
OS +0.25 –0.50 x 90

#5 (retinoscopy at 20 inches) OD +2.00 sph.
OS +2.25 –0.50 x 90

#7 (distance subjective) OD +0.75 -0.25 x 90
OS +0.25 sphere

#8 (distance phoria through #7)--3 exo
(Control at far, OU plano)

#9 (base out blur)--14

#10 (base-out break/recovery)--20 /4

#11 (base-in break/recovery)--8/5

#12 (distance vertical phoria)--Ortho

#13B (near phoria through #7)-1 exo

#14A (unfused cross cylinder) OD +2.50 -0.25 x 90
OS +2.25 sphere

#15A (phoria through #14A)--14 exo

#14B (fused cross cylinder) OD +2.00 -0.25 x 90
OS +1.75 sphere

#15B (phoria through #14B)--11 exo
(Control at near, OU plano)

#16A (base-out blur)--X   #16B (base-out break/recovery)--18/15

#17A (base-in blur)--13   #17B (base-in break/recovery)--19/16

#19 (binocular amplitude of accommodation)--3.75   (from #7)

#20 (minus lens to blur out)-- -1.00

#21 (plus lens to blur out)--+3.00

Stresspoint Retinoscope: OU +1.00 provided best balance

The same questions can and should be raised regarding Susan as were posed following the presentation of Brett's initial optometric examination earlier. Does Susan have a visual problem? What are her needs? Will an optometric program of care satisfy her needs? If so, what optometric program of care is appropriate?

The reader should attempt to answer the above questions with the foregoing information available. Susan's optometric data should be analyzed from your current perspective. If she was your patient, what would you recommend? What could you expect as a result of your recommendations? Can you predict the results? Can you analyze and diagnose the visual status from the behavioral point of view? How would an optometrist with a more classical concept of vision view Susan? And what would be the recommendation? If the data were analyzed from the viewpoint only of the Skeffington Analytical Method of Case Analysis using the seven directives for successful lens fitting, what would be the recommendations?

Hopefully, the reader will discipline himself and put himself through the above exercises, as this can be a most valuable learning experience.

STOP AND ANALYZE THE CASE

The reader was just introduced to Susan D, an 18-year-old college freshman, who was seen for her first optometric examination. The examination visit coincided with her winter vacation and it followed completion of her first semester at college. The initial college semester was disappointing, considering her prior high school performance, as demonstrated by her grades. It was suggested that she might have a visual problem. The results of the examination were revealed. The reader was requested to do his own evaluation, preferably from different points of view, and then answer basic questions as follows:

1. Does Susan haves a visual problem?
2. What are her needs?
3. Will an optometric program of care satisfy her needs?
4. What optometric program of care is appropriate?

Does Susan have a visual problem? Before answering this question, it is important to discuss the term, *visual problem*, as used within the behavioral concept framework. Then, it would be appropriate to answer the more fundamental question—what is a visual problem? As with other terminology (such as the word vision), the use and meaning of such terms vary depending on the model used by the optometrist.

Visual Problem: A visual problem is an unsatisfied vision-related personal need. The term is purposely "person-oriented" and it relates specifically to the identified and recognized visual needs of a person. A visual problem is person-oriented rather than measurement-oriented. The condition of the person's vision system is evaluated and appraised based on the observations, measurements and findings attained during the course of the optometric examination.

Visual Conditions: Remember the definition of optometry—the profession specializing in the examination, diagnosis and treatment of conditions of the vision system. Thus, conditions are measurement-oriented and directly relate to the physiology of the vision system. The condition may be such that, in the opinion of the optometrist, there is no identifiable clinical deviation to indicate impairment. On the other hand, the evaluation of the data may reveal physiological impairment or limitations in the vision system. If this is the case, the optometrist would conclude that a dysfunction or disability in the vision system exists and represents a condition that may require a treatment or program of care. Again, the importance of the concept of vision reveals itself because the identification of a condition varies from one point of view to another. Even the labels of conditions vary.

Visual Needs: The behavioral concept emphasizes the person and the NEEDS of the person. On the other hand, concepts other than the behavioral seem to be more measurement-oriented, i.e., the program of care is more dictated by what the optometrist sees in his findings rather than what he hears from his patient.

From the behavioral point of view, the following are conceivable:

1. The patient reveals an impaired condition but has no visual problem.
2. The patient has a visual problem but no evidence of dysfunction.

The vast majority of people with visual problems reveal evidences of physiological impairment, and the optometric goal is to provide a level of care to alleviate the visual problem. In other words, the goal is to satisfy the patient's needs. An excellent example of a patient with impairment but no visual problem will be shown later.

Case History and Needs

It is critical to emphasize the importance of the case history. This should be obvious. Frequently, the so-called chief complaint does not truly describe the real need or needs of any given patient. The behavior, visual demands and visual needs must be explored totally. Many patients have vision-oriented needs. Unless the optometrist explores these needs, the patient would never be aware that his or her needs are related to the adequacy of the vision system. Many people function at a level lower than desired in many vision-oriented activities and do not appreciate that the activity is vision-related, i.e., sports, reading, general job demands.

It is truly difficult to think of many non-vision demanding activities of human behavior. After all, the vision process is dominant in human behavior.

The case history must include an inventory of the significant critical vision demands of the patient as well as the patient's critique of how adequate the demands are being met. These are the needs descriptive of a patient's visual problem.

Does Susan have a visual problem? Yes.

What are her needs: They are as follows:

1. Freedom from tired and itchy eyes
2. Increased reading efficiency (speed and comprehension)
3. Eliminate re-reading for meaning
4. Increased ability to concentrate
5. Improvement in freedom to achieve at the college level

Will an optometric program of care satisfy her needs? Yes.

What optometric program of care is appropriate?

Before answering the final question, the examination data must be evaluated, appraised and the case diagnosed more specifically.

Visual Analysis

The findings of the analytical examination sequence reveal that Susan's visual behavior is partially embedded. There is no evidence of an early existing vision development problem. The performance observations of poor ocular motility and suppressions affirm that her information processing is restricted and limited. The poor quality of response monocularly on visual acuity is also a product of this limitation. Stresspoint retinoscopy reveals the availability of counter-stress lenses. Quoting the summation statement from the author's written notes on Susan:

> *The optometric evaluation of the collected data and information reveals the partially embedded syndrome of the stress-induced visual problem associated with reduced and restricted visual efficiency as a product of interference with information processing ability. Visual discomfort (tired and itching eyes) is expressed when the level of demand is greater than the freedom to meet the demand.*

It was conjectured that Susan's vision disability, a stress-induced visual problem, was created in elementary school years, probably between fourth and sixth grade. The mode of adaptation was reduced visual efficiency (the source of slow, effortful reading) and avoidance of excessive near-centered demands. She used her auditory processes to compensate for her disabilities. In other words, she became an auditory learner. This is not unusual. Many people with this type of disability can do very well in the average high school as an auditory learner, but not in college. Many of these visual dysfunctions do not make themselves known until the person comes face to face with college level demands and is forced to use the visual system in order to survive. Now faced with college demands, Susan, a person who was a high achiever in less demanding environments, is now acutely aware of her restrictions. The existence of some degree of discomfort suggests that she has tried to cope, but that the visual demands are greater than the freedom to meet such demands.

It is further conjectured that the visual behavior would have been significantly more embedded if she were seen before she began college. The present demands, however, have created additional excessive stress resulting in a less embedded pattern of behavior.

But what visual care does one recommend and what can be expected?

From a conventional point view, there are two possible approaches:

1. She has 20/20 acuity, healthy eyes and no ocular defects; therefore, do nothing.
2. Prescribe compensatory lenses equivalent to the #7 finding. If one approaches this, using the Skeffington Analytical Sequence and the seven directives of successful lens fitting, this is exactly what would be done. It is a "safe" and acceptable lens—but what benefits could really be anticipated?

Considering the degree of restriction and impairment imposed on Susan by this dysfunction, there is no question that a program of visual training is required to provide her with the opportunity to develop adequate visual abilities in order to satisfy her total needs. But, practicality must be considered. She is going to college in an area where there is no colleague to whom she could be referred for visual training. A complete "out-of-office" visual training program is questionable from the standpoint of practicality and its effectiveness in her situation is doubtful.

What, then, can be expected as a product of using lenses prescribed from the behavioral viewpoint? Which of her needs can be satisfied? The answers to these questions are quoted from the author's notes and are summarized as follows:

...provide appropriate counter-stress lenses in single vision form to be used for all near-centered demands. The use of such lenses will reduce current stress, providing increased comfort and comfort maintenance; increase sustaining ability on a near-centered task; and control and protect against possible additional adverse adaptation such as secondary myopia. In using these lenses, avoidance (of nearpoint tasks) may be reduced and minimal gains in visual efficiency realized if for no reason other than being able to sustain on a task more easily. Return for progress case study during spring vacation from college.

The above describes the extent of benefits expected as a result of using counter-stress lenses.

It was not expected, however, that the use of the lenses alone would alleviate the disability or satisfy all the identified needs. The value of the lenses is limited because of the degree of embeddedness. In reality, the use of such lenses will permit her to function more effectively within the framework of the existing condition. The lenses will be used initially as remedial lenses and they will enable her to gain as much as possible as a product of use. Ultimately, they will be utilized as controlling, protecting and maintenance lenses in order to permit her an opportunity to preserve her existing level of ability. Then, if available and desired, she can be considered for acceptance as a visual training patient for maximum benefits and satisfaction for all her needs.

The prescription was OU +1.00 spheres.

Progress Case Study: Reporting that she had been using the glasses properly, Susan returned for her progress case study three months later. No longer does she experience any form of discomfort and she feels more able to cope with college demands. Performances on quizzes and exams confirm these feelings. The optometric examination data is as follows:

Unaided visual acuity at far: Right, left and both eyes 20/20

Unaided visual acuity at near: Right, left and both eyes 20/20

Cover test: ortho far and near

Convergence nearpoint: 2 inches left eye deviates and reports diplopia, recovery at 4 inches

Ocular motility: pursuit movements full, spastic and jerky; fixations less erratic

The Analytical Examination Sequence:

#3 (habitual distance phoria)--½ exo

#4 (distance retinoscopy)   OU +0.50 spheres

#5 (retinoscopy at 20 inches)   OU +2.00 spheres

#7 (distance subjective)   OD +0.75 spheres
                                 OS +0.50 spheres

#8 (phoria through #7)--2 exo
   (Control at far: OU Plano)

#9 (base-out blur)--13

#10 (base-out break/recovery)--23/5

#11 (base-in break/recovery)--9/5
    (Control at near: OU +1.00 spheres)

#13A (habitual near phoria)--2 eso

#13B (near phoria through #7)--5 exo

#16A (base out blur)--X   #16B (base out break/recovery)--19/6

#17A (base in blur)--X   #17B (base in break/recovery)--24/16

Stresspoint Retinoscopy: OU +2.00 spheres provided best balance

Based on Susan's report, the predicted benefits are being realized (nothing more; nothing less). She was instructed to continue the same use of the lenses and to return for her next programmed progress case study at the end of summer prior to returning for her second year of college. She was told that the form of her lenses may be changed at that time to a dual focus lens with Plano uppers for her maximum convenience. And, once again, she was reminded that visual training would be available to her if she was had the time and desired benefits that could be gained. In the meantime, she certainly has benefited from the power of lenses.

Case Study: Mr. LK

Earlier, it was noted that a person could reveal vision dysfunction yet have no visual problem. The following is such a case. LK, age 38 years, presented himself for a complete optometric examination because it had been eight years since his last examination in another city and he thought his "eyes should be checked" at least periodically. He was not aware of any visual problems. He is an excellent example of an individual with a severe physiological dysfunction. Yet, he has no visual problem.

The case study is presented without further comment.

Case History: Has had prior examinations, the last time being nearly eight years ago. He has never had any glasses or recommendations for any form of vision care. He is a successful TV network news editor and does a lot of reading and other close work daily. He sees clearly at far and near and he reports no aspects of discomfort. He feels that he is a fast and efficient reader (he has to be on his job). He experiences no undue fatigue and he reports no problem with space judgments. He plays tennis well and he is not aware of any restrictions. He is satisfied with his game.

The investigation of eye health status revealed the eyes and adnexa to be free from pathology and abnormality.

The Optometric Examination:

Unaided visual acuity at far: Right slow 20/20; Left 20/40; Both eyes 20/20-

Unaided visual acuity at near: Right 20/20; Left 20/30-; Both eyes 20/20

Cover test: exophoria far and near

Convergence nearpoint: 8 inches, right eye deviates and reports diplopia, recovery at 11 inches

Ocular motility: both pursuit and fixation movements extremely poor, spastic and erratic

Visual Abilities: (Telebinocular, DB series)

    DB 10 (pig and dog): both present in exo position
    DB 8 (line and ball): suppression
    DB4K (3-4 ball test far): 4 balls in exo position
    DB6D (stereopsis): #11
    BU21 (stereo/suppression test): patient suppressed
    DB3 and DB2 (signboards): 20/20
    DB9 (far) (arrow and numbers): #10
    DB9 (near) (arrow and numbers): #6 ½
    DB5K (3-4 ball test near): 4 balls in exo

Wirt Stereo: 9

The Analytical Examination

#3(distance habitual phoria)--10 exo #13A (near habitual phoria)--14 exo

#4 (retinoscopy)--OU -0.50 spheres

#5 (retinoscopy at 20 inches) OD +1.50 -0.75 x 25
OS +1.50 -0.75 x 70

#7 (subjective) OD Plano -0.50 x 105
OS +0.25 -1.25 x 90

#8 (phoria through #7)--9 exo
   (Control at far: #7)

#9 (base out blur)--X   #10 (base out break/recovery)--9/-3

#11 (base in break/recovery)--10/7

#12 (vertical phoria)--Ortho phoria

#13B (near phoria through #7)--16 exo

#14A (unfused cross cylinder) OD Plano -0.50 x 105
OS +0.75 -1.25 x 90

#15A (phoria through #14A)--16 exo

#14B (fused cross cylinder)--same as #14A

#15B (phoria through #14B)--18 exo
   (Control at near: #7)

#16A (base out blur)--X   #16B (base out break/recovery)--5/-6

#17A (base in blur)--X   #17B (base in break/recovery)--19/17

#19 (binocular amplitude of accommodation)--3.75

#20 (minus lens to blur out)-- -3.00

#21 (plus lens to blur out)--+2.75

Summation statements regarding L. K. were as follows:
The optometric evaluation of the collected data and information reveals the embedded syndrome of the stress-induced visual problem with the adaptation of divergence excess and intermittent divergent strabismus. Apparently, adequate adaptation has been made since he has been free of both awareness and symptoms that might have been resulting from this disability.

CHAPTER 4
Preventive Optometric Care

It has been emphasized throughout these chapters that the meaning of different words will vary frequently and depend on the user's point of view or concept. One may use a specific word in communication with full knowledge as to the word's meaning—that is, to the user. But, the receiver hears or reads the word in terms meaningful to the receiver. When this occurs, there may be no communication.

In recognition of this potential communication gap, the author has specifically defined words and terms used by the author that may be common to the profession yet vary in meaning, depending on the concept from which it is viewed.

An example of this is a rather commonly used word and a common term in the health care professions, including optometry. The word is *prevention* and the term is *preventive care*. Pause for a moment and ponder. What do these mean to you in general? What do they mean to you as an optometrist? What does the word prevention and the term preventive care mean to your optometric patients?

The dictionary defines prevention as "the action of overtaking or anticipating." Likewise, preventive medicine (Webster's Unabridged Dictionary) is defined as "a branch of medical science dealing with methods of preventing the occurrence of disease." Although it is not in the dictionary, preventive optometry may be defined as "that aspect of optometry dealing with methods of preventing the occurrence of dysfunction of the vision system."

Although the dictionary definitions are specific as to the meanings of prevention and preventive care, it is interesting to note that the health care fields use these terms frequently to mean early identification of deviancy from the unimpaired. This is unfortunate and it has led to some degree of confusion. Literally, prevention is dealing with something before the fact, whereas early identification, important as it is, is dealing with something after the fact. Early identification of impairment is significant itself. Within the corpus of behavioral optometry; it would imply the identification of vision dysfunction at an early stage. As an example, this might be the case of non-embedded behavior. But, this is not prevention in that a disability is already observed.

Within optometry (the discipline of vision) prevention and preventive vision care have meaning only when the visual process is viewed from the behavioral model. An inspection of all other concepts of vision and vision care will reveal that there is no consideration of preventive care. Any consideration of prevention must be related of necessity to etiological concepts. Regarding other concepts of vision the etiology assumed of dysfunction may either be genetic, a physical abnormality or simply fatalistic. Accommodative-convergence models give no insight at all to etiology. The implication is that the disability is just a part of the person. It is impossible for prevention to enter into clinical involvement if the optometrist applies this concept in an attitude towards patients. It is within this scope of optometric practice, however, where the term preventive care frequently has been used to mean early identification and, therefore, early intervention.

The fundamental tenets of the behavioral concept were stated in Chapter 1. Refer to tenets number 2 and number 5. Based on empirical experience and clinical observation, the position is taken that vision is developed and that vision dysfunction is an alteration in the normal development or developed process of vision. If this is true, the implication is that one cannot be conceived with a vision disability or born with a dysfunction. It is conceivable that an infant can emerge into the world with inadequate physical equipment, the extreme being born without eyes. But, even in this situation the vision impairment is the result of inadequate development due to defective structure delimiting the developing process. If vision is developed it is a product of physiological learning or adaptation resulting from appropriate experiences being impinged on a maturationally-ready system within the environment of the individual. And, finally, if vision is developed the developing process can be interfered with or that which has been developed can be interfered with, resulting in an impaired vision condition or maladaptation.

This is the underlying notion that permits the rationale for visual training. Thus, if vision is developed, the process can be enhanced and visual dysfunction is alleviated by way of replacement of impaired performance patterns with more effective, efficient, and economical movement patterns.

The principle to be derived from this information and these statements is that impaired vision conditions are the result of environmental influences. Given this, environmental factors can and should be controlled—hence, the reality of the notion of prevention of visual dysfunction and preventive optometric care.

When vision development is thwarted the result, observed clinically, is a vision development problem. Clinical manifestations of vision development problems include strabismus, amblyopia, extreme myopia, the excessive amounts of astigmatism (particularly monocular) seen in the preschool-aged, adverse hyperopia, and the most common (for lack of an adequate label), the visually-unready child. These are the vision conditions resulting from interference in the developing process of vision.

Actually, a vision development problem reflects a child development problem viewed optometrically and it requires optometric care. (A full consideration of this topic, however, goes beyond the extent of these chapters and the reader should refer to other OEP Foundation chapters devoted to developmental vision.) Suffice it to say that the thwarting in the developing process is the result of restriction, restraint and/or deprivation imposed on the developing child that would be evidenced during the first five or six years of life. Fortunately, no greater than 20% of all impaired vision conditions are of this type. Preventive optometric care as it relates to vision development is primarily that of appropriate parental guidance. The importance of arranging and providing adequate opportunities for development and on how to avoid conditions which may thwart development are stressed. (Again, for detailed insight, the reader is referred to the abundance of literature on this topic available from the OEP Foundation.)

Clinical evidence has revealed that the vast majority of dysfunctions of the vision system arise after the child has reached school age and has been exposed to the standard academic environment. Probably the most elaborate study, as well as the most famous, was the 1942-48 Texas Project (Darell Boyd Harmon, Ph.D., Director of the Texas State Health Department).[1] This was not an optometric study, nor was it primarily a vision study.

Involving 160,000 school-aged children, it was a longitudinal study of the learning environment and its influence on the physiology and physical attributes of the child. Visual behavior was only one aspect studied. This investigation revealed that nearly 20% of children entering first grade demonstrated visual dysfunction. This figure doubled by the third to fourth grade and redoubled by fifth to sixth grade. Undoubtedly, the study revealed the high incidence of impaired vision conditions and that impairments within a population increased as the child moved along within the demands of the academic environment.

A significant fact, which still today is not widely known, was revealed by the investigation. The study reported that approximately 80% of the population demonstrated an impaired vision condition by the latter part of elementary school. Yet, it was conjectured that at least half of this group could have gone many years without being aware of any visual dysfunction. The Texas Project led Harmon to conclude that the prime stressor agent responsible for impairment in visual function was the biologically unacceptable, visually-compulsive near-centered task.

Assuming that a significant portion of the 20% of children entering first grade with vision dysfunction are etiologically vision development problems, it would be logical to conclude that the vast majority of the increased incidence of disabilities identified with increasing academic years represent stress-induced visual problems. The term used years ago to describe this syndrome was nearpoint visual problems. These are impaired vision conditions resulting from interference in the developed process of vision. The provoking stressor agent is near-centered demand which induces stress within the vision system. The organism responds to this stress and it begins the process of adaptation (maladaptation, actually), a factor of time. The initial response to the stressor agent is described as the non-embedded syndrome immediately beginning the movement in time toward embedded behavior. There are two general avenues of adaptation along which the impaired individual moves. Some people adapt along the avenue of myopia but the majority develop the syndrome of reduced visual efficiency.

The optometric appreciation of the etiology of the stress-induced visual problem provides great opportunity for optometry to demonstrate its uniqueness and, in particular, preventive optometric care. If the stress-induced dysfunction is a product of the environment, can the stressor agent be alleviated or reduced so that stress-induced problems may be prevented?

We cannot eliminate the academic environment since it is a part of our culture. That is, we cannot remove the demands imposed by the near-centered task. But, can we arrange conditions to permit a person to better meet the imposed demands without adverse effect? The answer is "yes." How? We do this by using lenses. Herein lies the most significant value of counter-stress lenses and, more specifically, convex lenses referred to frequently as "low power" lenses. When should these lenses be provided and how is the prescription determined? These are the most important questions.

Some believed idealistically years ago that all children should enter first grade with preventive plus lenses. We promoted this idea and sent many children to first grade with their preventive lenses. But frequently the outcome was disappointing. Visual problems were not totally prevented. Obviously this was not the answer. With additional clinical experience it was realized that the value of stress-relieving lenses was not to be disputed. But, it could not be "shot- gunned." There is a right time. There are specifically determined prescriptions appropriate for each and every child. But, the child must be viewed as an individual and dealt with as such. Sooner or later as the child grows he reaches a point in time as a product of development where it can be demonstrated that he is vulnerable to stress induced by the near-centered task. It is at this time that the preventive lenses are initially significant. This is not to say that the child will immediately induce dysfunction if he is not provided with preventive lenses at the time of vulnerability. But, he is vulnerable. The chances are great that such a problem sooner or later would emerge if preventive lenses are not supplied.

However, it must be appreciated that prevention, actually, is the hardest thing to sell in any field or area. It is easy to talk about and it is fascinating to discuss. Yet, it is frequently difficult to accept. Consider the emotional difficulty of parents who are told that their child's visual process is free of impairment yet he/she requires glasses. Glasses have long been considered an undesired necessity when something is wrong. Now, we want to prescribe glasses when and because all is right. From a practice management point of view this must be handled very carefully and judiciously.

Parents must be educated and oriented to the notion of prevention so that, when the time comes for the initial recommendation for preventive lenses, it is accepted and appreciated. Parents must assume an attitude of pride in being able to permit their child the opportunity to prevent dysfunction and prevent problems for which the parents, perhaps, never had the opportunity. Parents must be prepared to defend their child's right to prevent a problem. The author prescribes preventive lenses only if these conditions are met.

Finally, the question as to the means of determining the need for preventive lenses and how to determine the specific prescription must be broached. For more than 20 years, the author has relied on the stresspoint retinoscope technique and measurement for this information and insight.

Reference
1. Harmon DB. The Co-ordinated Classroom: A Monograph. American Seating Co. 1949.

CHAPTER 5
Stresspoint Retinoscopy

Optometry believes that only through the application of the unique optometric understanding of the role of lenses to the biological demands, and the needs and methodology of the arranged conditions for learning, can any individual living in our modern culture attain anywhere near the size and stature of his inherent endowment and capacities.

Optometry believes that the one and only completely proper lens is the one that will most nearly satisfy the avoidance reaction produced by the organismic response to containment.

Optometry holds that this determination of the optimal lens is not covariant with the measurement of the refractive status of the eye but is determined by the clinical understanding of the problem.

These statements by the late A. M. Skeffington, O.D., former Director of Education for the Optometric Extension Program Foundation, are as meaningful and significant for the behavioral optometrist today as when they were made in the 1960's. Dr. Skeffington's thoughts are the essence of these chapters. They represent the core of the *Behavioral Concept of Vision*.

Skeffington always said that the fundamental role of the optometrist is to fit a pair of lenses. Ultimately, this led to the creation and development of the Skeffington Analytical Sequence. Skeffington was asked in later years about stress-relieving lenses for preventive purposes. "Would you put lenses on every child?" he was asked. Skeffington would answer, "Would you protect the learning ability of every child?" If the original question had been, "Would you put lenses on everyone?" then, perhaps, the appropriate answer would have been another question, "Would you protect the learning and earning ability of everyone?"

If, as Skeffington stated, "the optimal lens is not covariant with the measurement of the refractive status of the eye ...," then the fundamental question that is answered by this chapter is, "How does the optometrist determine the optimal lens formula that will provide the benefits of prevention, protection, maintenance, remediation and enhancement of visual performance as required and desired by any given patient?"

The determination and utilization of such lenses is not new. Skeffington's comments are a couple of generations old but the inherent notions and applications are even older. Historically, the optometrist providing a behavioral approach to vision care long sought the ways and means to define and refine the determination of the optimal lens formula in terms of optometric method. Such a determination varied from sheer judgment to subjective (patient feeling tone) to objective means.

The search has been on to determine a method that optimally would provide the appropriate information, be consistent and repeatable, and be taught easily and accepted within the capacity of the average optometrist.

Contrary to what has been assumed mistakenly such a lens value is NOT determined from the collected data of the analytical examination. Nor should this be presumed as the lens formula evidenced in the seven directives for successful lens fitting. After all, the latter is the determination of a lens formula that a patient will wear. Frequently, this has been referred to as the "safe" lens. Although the lens value for optimal performance is not determined or found within the analytical findings, appropriate interpretation of these findings determines the value of the optimal lens formula to the patient.

The optimal lens referred to by Skeffington has been labeled more commonly as the counter-stress or stress-relieving lens. Numerous procedures for such determination have emerged over the years, as suggested earlier, such as the Macdonald Form Field Technique (a subjective procedure) and other more objective methods primarily taking advantage of the retinoscope. Examples of these are book retinoscopy (Getman), MEM retinoscopy (Haynes), bell retinoscopy (Henry, Streff and Apell) and stresspoint retinoscopy. The latter, stresspoint retinoscopy, has been the procedure relied on by the author for more than 20 years to make this determination. The author is convinced that this procedure is the only means, presently known, to make this determination directly and specifically. All other techniques rely on professional judgment and patient subjectivity or, they are indirect determinants of that which stresspoint retinoscopy directly provides.

Stresspoint Retinoscopy

D. B. Harmon, Ph.D., directed research in the late 1950's at the Neurological Institute in Austin, Texas. His research included the filmed electromyographic and lens studies. Harmon noted and demonstrated at the time of those investigations that some interesting physiological changes took place when the target, approaching the subject with the subject fixating the target, was a certain distance from the subject. It was noted with a spot retinoscope used for observation that the brightness of the reflex changes. At first it brightens, immediately followed by a dulling and then followed by a return to the prior level of brightness. There was also a simultaneous flattening of the pulse pressure as well as an observable inner canthi twitch. It seemed that this was a significant point of measurement and it was, in fact, a measurement of a stress point. That is, it was an observation of the distance of near fixation where the person was confronted by the stress of close fixation and was forced to react, i.e., fight or flight.

It was concluded after personal discussion with Dr. Harmon that this method of observation and its application might provide a quantitative means to determine directly the counter-stress lens formula. It was apparent, after all, that lenses influenced this stress point. Plus lenses tended to cause this reaction to occur with fixation closer, minus lenses removed the stress point away further.

Obviously, it would be desirable to have the stress point closer than the person's normal working near distance. Harmon determined both physiologically and empirically that it would be desirable to have this stress point in children occur for best balance approximately 4 inches closer than the working distance.

This author routinely has done "stresspoint retinoscopy" on all patients since 1959 in order to compare the relationship between the counter-stress lenses demonstrated by this method with the lenses demonstrated by prior empirical qualitative means. Adequate skills and confidence resulted from the use of this procedure after many observations and conclusions (and due time). And now the author uses it as the prime determinant of the optimal lens formula.

The clinical procedure for stresspoint retinoscopy

The patient is seated in the examining chair. The retinoscope is held 20 inches away at a fixed position. The fixation target, the dangled bell, is held at the level of the retinoscope with the patient's attention directed to fixate on the bell as it is gradually moved toward the patient on midline. Both reflex motion and brightness are observed and noted as distance changes. This is observed first without lenses and/or with habitual lenses. Then, appropriate equal plus or minus spheres are added and observations repeated. The added lenses which shift the stress point to the desired position represent the acceptable counter-stress lens formula. Once again, it must be emphasized that the significance of these lenses is determined as a product of the insight derived from an analysis of the analytical examination data.

Some salient comments and observations

1. The stress point is organismic. That is, it is a bilateral response of the total person observed conveniently with the aid of a retinoscope. Thus, the occurrence of the stress point will be observed in either eye simultaneously. The position of the stress point will be generally the same for either eye with the exception of embedded asymmetric behavior accompanied by measurable anisometropia.

2. Although it was initially suggested that the stress point for children should be about 4 inches closer than the balanced working distance, experience has revealed even more definitive guidelines. This seems to hold true in the case of youngsters. But, as youngsters grow to young adults and then adults, it becomes more common to find and establish the stress point for best control and balance at a distance between 8 and 9 inches from the face. In other words, the more adult the individual, the more space needed between working distance and the stress point.

3. Frequently, it may be noted that two or three different pairs of lenses may shift the stress point to the approximate desired position. Clinical experience reveals that the desired pair is that with the brightest initial reflex. If three pairs of lenses have the same brightness, use the middle pair. If two pair are equal, split the means. In other words, use plus .62D if the lenses used are a pair of plus .50D and a pair of plus .75D—each equally bright with the stress point at the desired position.

4. Ultimately approaching the so-called Harmon distance (best balanced working near distance equivalent to distance measured from middle knuckle to elbow), clinical experience reveals that the stress point recedes from the face as the child grows. For example, the stress point in preschool-aged children is near the face. It may be 3 inches away when the child is age 3, and 4 inches away when the same child is seen a year later. This insight is extremely significant when consideration is given to the use of lenses for preventive purposes. This sets guidelines as to when a child should be provided with initial preventive counter-stress lenses. The rule is that the child is vulnerable to stress imposed by product of containment and ready for preventive lenses when the stress point is nearer than 4 inches to the child's "Harmon distance" and when the child is in a socially demanding near-centered environment. Clinically, it is known that the vast majority of children reach this time of vulnerability between the ages of 8 ½ and 11 years. However, some become vulnerable at earlier ages and others do not demonstrate any need for preventive lenses until the later teen years. This author still

has never seen anyone who did not demonstrate ultimately that preventive lenses would be needed sooner or later.

5. Generally speaking the stress point moves closer to the face as plus lenses are added. Adding plus continuously in most people will bring about a reversal eventually, and the stress point will seem to recede dramatically from the face. The more embedded the behavior the less plus that can be added before bringing about a reversal. The fully embedded emmetropic behavior will show the response reversal with as low a plus as a quarter of a diopter or an eighth of a diopter. Undoubtedly, this demonstrates the lack of acceptance of any lens power as well as the lack of value or acceptability of any lens power.

6. The initial retinoscopic observation may demonstrate "with" motion or "against" motion with patient fixating the target at 20 inches. Usually, the motion will be "against" when fixating at the 20-inch distance with the appropriate counter-stress lenses in place.

7. Compared to the bell retinoscopy procedure experience suggests the results of lens power indications are comparable. If there would be a difference, it would be expected that the bell retinoscopy procedure would show less plus than stresspoint retinoscopy. Appreciation of body dynamics would reveal that it is always safer to use less rather than excessive plus power if there had to be a variance from the ideal plus lens power. Although bell retinoscopy preceded stresspoint retinoscopy by many years, it purports to measure indirectly what stresspoint retinoscopy reveals directly.

8. There have been numerous cases observed wherein fixation on midline under habitual conditions showed an asymmetry. However, symmetry was brought about when equal plus lenses were applied. These were non-embedded behaviors. On the other hand, when the asymmetry was maintained, it was necessary to use the indicated difference in lens powers between the two eyes to provide the necessary counter-stress lenses as revealed by the stresspoint retinoscopy. These, of course, were more embedded behaviors.

9. The primary training lenses for formalized visual training are those indicated by stresspoint retinoscopy. As progression takes place in visual training the need to alter or modify the training lenses is determined by periodic monitoring via this procedure.

10. From a practical point of view, the author has found it convenient to have an assortment of "flipper" lenses available for use in stresspoint retinoscopy. The patient can hold the desired pair of lenses comfort-

ably in front of his eyes as the optometrist observes with the retinoscope in one hand and the fixation target in the other. The pairs of lenses are half diopter differences, i.e., one pair of plus .50D with the flip side being plus 1.00D. The author uses the following pairs: (a) OU +.50 and OU +1.00; (b) OU +.75 and OU +1.25; (c) OU +1.50 and OU +2.00; (d) OU -.50 and OU -1.00; and (e) OU -.75 and OU -1.25. Additional values can be derived through a combination of two flipper pairs. A tape measure or yardstick can be used to measure the distance from the patient. The distances are easily estimated after adequate practice.

The cases used in previous chapters to demonstrate the power of lenses have shown that the prescribed lenses are derived from the stresspoint retinoscopic technique. The following features an example of a patient revealing no lens value available, as well as one patient requiring the use of lenses solely for preventive purposes.

A Case Study

Susan R, age 24, was seen for her initial complete optometric examination by this author two years ago. She had had no prior vision care.

Susan had completed two years of college and then she had worked in an office. She had just recently started a more demanding desk-centered position. Generally, she saw clearly but she was aware of a delay in seeing clearly across the room after she did near-centered work. She reported symptoms of periodic diplopia and undue fatigue. Susan knew that she was a slow reader. Reading was tedious for her and it was not unusual for her to lose her place periodically. She had to reread for meaning. Spelling had never been one of her strengths.

The investigation of eye health status revealed that the eyes and adnexa were free of pathology and abnormality.

The data gathered from the optometric examination follows:

Unaided visual acuity at far and near: 20/20, right, left and both

Cover test: ortho at far, exophoria at near

Convergence nearpoint: 4 inches, right eye deviating outward and diplopia reported; recovery at eight inches

Ocular motility: pursuit movements were full and fairly smooth; fixations were accurate

Visual Abilities (Telebinocular, DB Series)

DB 10 (pig and dog): suppression
DB 8 (line and ball): suppression
DB4K (3 balls): 3 balls, suppression
DB6D (stereopsis): #12
BU21: (stereo/suppression test) patient suppressed
DB3 and DB2 (Signboards): 20/15
DB9 (far) (arrow and numbers): #9
DB9 (near)(arrow and numbers): #6
DB5K (3 balls at near): 4 balls in exo

Wirt Stereo: #9

The Analytical Examination:

#2 (keratometry)--OU sphere 44.25

#3 (distance habitual phoria)--4 exo   #13A (near habitual phoria)--9 exo

#4 (retinoscopy)   OD +0.25 sphere
                            OS +0.50 sphere

#5 (retinoscopy at 20 inches)--OU +2.00 sphere

#7 (subjective)   OD Plano
                            OS -0.25 x 60

#8 (phoria through #7)--4 exo

#9 (base out blur)--X

#10 (base out break/recovery)--13/8

#11 (base in break/recovery)--8/5

#13B (phoria at near through #7)--9 exo

#14A (unfused cross cylinder)   OD -0.25
                                OS -0.75 -0.25 x 60

#15A (phoria through #14A)--8 exo

#14B (fused cross cylinder)--same as #14A

#15B (phoria through #14B)--8 exo
    (control at near OU Plano)

#16A (base out blur)--X   #16B (base out break/recovery)--13/4

#17A (base in blur)--18   #17B (base in break/recovery)--24/16

#19 (binocular amplitude of accommodation)--7.50

#20 (minus lens to blur out)-- -4.00

#21 (plus lens to blur)--+0.50

Stresspoint Retinoscopy

Lenses used	Stresspoint
OU Plano	7 inches
OU +0.25 sphere	7 inches
OU +0.50 sphere	8 inches

An analysis of the collected data and information reveals the embedded syndrome of the stress-induced visual problem associated with reduced and restricted visual efficiency. There is no evidence of a vision development problem. Susan's symptoms suggest the levels of demand are greater than her freedom to meet the demands.

The Skeffington Analytical Sequence method of case analysis would reveal a deteriorated B1 and C type case. The seven directives of successful lens fitting would indicate that plus must be cut at all points since base-out findings at both far and near are low.

Since there is no plus at far and there is minus projection at near, there is no plus to "cut." In fact, there is no prescription of "safe" lenses that could be recommended to the patient according to this point of view. Anyone familiar with the deteriorating stages of a B and/or C type case would recognize that the only acceptable recommendation would be visual training.

The behavioral point of view suggests that this is an example of the embedded syndrome. Stresspoint retinoscopy demonstrates conclusively that there is no counter-stress lens formula available or even acceptable. The stress point is significantly closer than the balanced working distance. Plus 0.25 spheres do not shift the stress point, but plus 0.50 spheres bring about a reversal and it shifts the stress point further from the face.

Let us raise the four basic questions:

1. Does Miss Susan R have a visual problem? Yes.
2. What are her needs? Comfort, improved efficiency and increased freedom to perform.
3. Will an optometric program of care satisfy her needs? Yes.
4. What optometric program of care is appropriate? Visual training.

This is and will be the only case study presented in these chapters in which lenses alone will not be of value, acceptable or even conceivably prescribable. It was presented deliberately to demonstrate several points.

Alternatives of Care

The author prefers to offer each and every patient three alternatives of optometric care, sometimes referred to as good, better and best. The occasion arises in few cases when there are no significant alternatives available. This case study represents one of those infrequent occurrences.

Alternative #1 (good) is the offering of a lens formula based on the Skeffington Analytical Sequence method of case analysis and the application of the seven directives for successful lens fitting. This is the safe lens prescription that is acceptable and worn by any patient—assuming such a prescription is identifiable. Most commonly this is a compensatory prescription. It would be similar, if not equivalent, to a lens formula derived by the graphical and/or AC/A approach. There are occasions, of course, when the safe lens prescription is actually Plano, or no Rx.

Alternative #2 (better) is the recommendation of a pair of glasses that will provide the patient with benefits beyond those expected as a product of the #1 alternative. The prescription of lenses derived for alternative #2 is what these chapters are all about. It is indicative of the power of lenses. Depending on the patient's need and predictability of behavior, this lens formula provides benefits beyond compensation that may prevent, protect, maintain, remedy and/or enhance visual performance. If nothing else, it will be representative at least of the prescription determined to be acceptable and desirable by stresspoint retinoscopy. Thus, alternatives #1 and #2 are lens prescriptions, but they are significantly different prescriptions for different purposes and different levels of anticipated benefits.

Alternative #3 (best) is always formalized visual training and, for all practical purposes, every patient is offered this opportunity. It is only by means of visual training that one may have the privilege and the opportunity to develop and cultivate maximum levels of visual ability and derive maximum benefits. However, not everyone has needs that require formalized visual training. But, in the opinion of this author, the patient should be given the privilege.

The patient must have expressed needs to be accepted for visual training that can be satisfied only by developing more efficient and effective visual performance. If the expressed needs can be satisfied in a more simple approach, the patient is unacceptable for visual training. This author's attitude is based on the recognition that every human being can learn to see more efficiently but not everyone has to see more efficiently.

Susan R's visual behavior represented an infrequent occurrence in that there were no alternatives available. Alternative #1 was not available. The directives of successful lens fitting revealed no prescribable safe lens formula. Stresspoint retinoscopy demonstrated no available or acceptable counter-stress lens formula. Thus, there was no alternative #2. The behavior was too embedded. Yet, the patient had legitimate needs that could be satisfied only by an optometric program of care and, in her case, the only recommendation was visual training. If there was an alternative, albeit most unsatisfactory, it would have been to alter her lifestyle and reduce the demand level.

Fortunately, she chose the more positive approach—visual training—that enabled her to maintain her lifestyle, increase her ability to meet the higher level demands and develop the freedom to function at heights greater than she had ever conceived. No other discipline—no other approach in vision care—could provide this opportunity. Only the optometrist who appreciates the behavioral concept could offer such an opportunity.

The case data demonstrate the reliability of the basic Skeffington Analytical Sequence method of case analysis and the value of the seven directives for successful lens fitting. By following the directives the optometrist would recognize, if nothing else, that he could not alleviate the patient's symptoms with any pair of glasses. From the behavioral point of view, the case data represent a very embedded visual behavior and the stresspoint retinoscopy further substantiates the fact that no lens approach is available. In fact, the reversal response, as demonstrated with the stresspoint retinoscopy, provides additional evidence of the reliability of the embedded syndrome as well as the validity of the Behavioral Concept of Vision.

Another Case Study

The following case study is presented in contrast and to exemplify preventive optometry peculiar to the behavioral approach. John David C, age 4 ½, was seen in May for his first complete optometric examination. At the time, there were no symptoms or parental observations to suggest vision dysfunction. In response to the question raised on the developmental history questionnaire, "Why do you think your child needs a visual examination?" the parents wrote, "for preventive reasons." John David's parents were both patients and had been made aware of the importance of early child optometric examinations and preventive care. Ideally, it would have been more desirable to have begun his optometric care at an earlier age.

He was enrolled at the time in a Montessori preschool program (and doing very well). Without going into complete detail, the results gleaned from his first optometric investigation were as follows:

1. There was no evidence of any ocular pathology or abnormality.

2. There was no evidence of ocular defect or interference in vision development.
3. Unaided visual acuity at far and near was 20/20 right, left and both eyes.
4. General performance suggested good developmental processes as a result of an obviously excellent developmental opportunity.
5. Movement coordination, in relationship to the task demands, seemed to be the major weak area of performance and may need some encouragement.
6. Stresspoint retinoscopy—the stress point was at 4 inches; there was no need or reason to shift it at this time.

The summation and recommendations as reported to the parents were as follows:

The optometric evaluation of the collected data and information reveals no evidence of a vision development problem. However, there are some warning signals. Generally speaking, boys develop 20/20 (distance and near) visual acuity between 5 ½ and 6 ½ years. Early development of 20/20 in boys is frequently associated with later myopia development and usually relates to weakness in motor coordination development. These two aspects exist now and may be the warning signal for later change in visual function. Therefore, it is recommended that particular emphasis be placed on motor coordination development by means of specific activities to be done at home as well as encouraged in the preschool program.

The parents were provided with a copy of G. N. Getman's book, *How to Develop Your Child's Intelligence*, with specific recommended activities to be done noted.

The child was programmed to be seen next for a complete reevaluation in one year.

John David returned the following May for his annual examination. There was no evidence of any dysfunction in the visual process, but it was recommended that he continue with movement coordination activities. The stress point was still at 4 inches and no lenses were recommended or required. He was programmed once again to return in one year for reexamination. The results were similar the following May. The stress point shifted to 5 inches and once again, no lenses were recommended. The one-year programming was maintained.

John David was seen again in late May of the next year. He was completing second grade in a parochial school and he was doing very well with general movement coordination reported excellent. No ocular defects were noted. However, pursuit movements were spastic. Slight suppression was revealed on Telebinocular tests and the analytical demonstrated an apparent non-embedded syndrome, which could reflect an early stage stress-induced visual problem. He held reading material at an 8 inches distance although his Harmon distance was 10 inches.

Stresspoint retinoscopy was as follows: stress point without lenses at 8 inches; with plus 0.75D at 6 inches; with plus 1.25D at 10 inches. It was indicated that counter-stress lenses could immediately be provided. However, lenses were not provided yet because it was nearly the end of the school year. He would be permitted to have a summer free of stress with much outdoor activity. He would be reappraised in September at the beginning of the school year. Of course, it was noted that he might have need of counter-stress lenses in the fall.

There was no evidence of dysfunction in September. No longer did there exist an apparent non-embedded syndrome. The stress point without any lenses was at 6 inches, his Harmon distance being 10 inches. With plus 0.75D, stress point was also at 6 inches. The indications were that preventive counter-stress lenses still were not required. It was recommended that he be seen again in six months (the following March) because of what was seen the previous May.

As programmed, John David returned for the recommended reexamination in March. Once again, performance in all areas was reported as being excellent. He had no symptoms, nor was there any parental observations suggesting visual dysfunction. The examination revealed no evidence of a stress-induced visual problem. However, the stress point without lenses was at 9 inches, with plus 0.75D at 6 inches and with plus 1.25D at 4 inches. Prior professional experience indicated that John David was definitely vulnerable to the stresses imposed by containment and for the purpose of pure prevention was now ready for stress-relieving lenses. Obviously, both his parents and John David had been adequately prepared for this "momentous" occasion. They agreed and accepted the notion of such lenses for all near-centered activities, not because anything was wrong, but rather to keep it right and to prevent any visual dysfunction and visual problem. He was given OU Plano, add 0.75 in executive bifocals, the segment height placed at the level of the lower edge of pupils. His next scheduled appointment was arranged for July.

The progress case study appointment in July revealed no evidence of any problems. Lenses had been properly used and the stress points were identical. He was instructed to continue the use of the preventive lenses and to return the following May when he would near the end of fourth grade. Again, lenses had been properly used, no problems revealed and he was programmed once more on an annual basis.

John David has been programmed annually since that May 1974. As of this writing, his most recent office visit was in April 1981. He is now 16 years old, in 11th grade, a superb student and athlete, a karate expert and instructor. He has continued to use his preventive lenses faithfully for all near-centered demands. The prescription has never needed to be altered. Obviously, the size of the glasses had to be modified two or three times because of John David's normal growth. The following represents the stresspoint retinoscopy observations over the years, beginning with the first May findings:

Stress Point	Without Lenses (inches)	With +0.75 (inches)
5/4/74	11	7
5/24/75	11	7
6/15/76	10	6
8/9/77	13	8
12/2/78	13	8
3/8/80	14	8
4/4/81	14	8

To complete the story of John David, the data from his most recent optometric examination is provided.

Unaided visual acuity at far and near: 20/20 right, left and both

Cover test: ortho at far and near

Convergence nearpoint: one inch, left eye deviating outward and diplopia reported; recovery at four inches

Ocular motility: pursuit movements full and smooth; fixations accurate

Visual abilities (Telebinocular, DB Series)

    DB10 (pig and dog): present, no suppression
    DB 8 (line and ball): line seen through ball, no suppression
    DB4K (3 balls): 3 balls, no suppression
    DB6D (stereopsis): #12
    DB3 and DB3 (signboards): 20/17   DB9 (far) (arrow and numbers): #9, steady
    DB9 (near) (arrow and numbers): #4 ½, steady
    DB5K (3 balls at near): 3 balls, no suppression

Wirt Stereo: #9   Randot: #8

The Analytical Examination

#3 (distance habitual phoria)--1 eso   #13A (near habitual phoria)--½ eso

#4 (retinoscopy)--OU -0.25 sphere

#5 (retinoscopy at 20 inches)--OU +1.50 sphere

#7 (subjective)--OU +0.50 sphere

#8 (phoria through #7)--1 eso

#9 (base out blur)--X

#10 (base out break/recovery)--16/7

#11 (base in break/recovery)--7/3

#13B (near phoria through #7)--3 exo

#14A (unfused cross cylinder)--OU +1.50

#15A (phoria through #14A)--5 exo

#14B (fused cross cylinder)--OU +1.00

#15B (phoria through #14B)--2 exo
    (control at near OU +0.75 sphere)

#16A (base out blur)--X   #16B (base out break/recovery)--19/8

#17A (base in blur)--X   #17B (base in break/recovery)--20/11

#19 (binocular amplitude of accommodation)--6.00

#20 (minus lens to blur out)-- -2.75

#21 (plus lens to blur out)-- +1.75

CHAPTER 6
The Visual Process

A. M. Skeffington, O.D., claimed that the value of a lens is that it could change orders to the system. In other words, he suggested that the final response of an organism differed as input was altered and programming changed. Samuel Renshaw, Ph.D., professor of experimental psychology, Ohio State University, always insisted that the stimulus lies within the act rather than outside the act. From this was derived Renshaw's oft-quoted statement that "seeing is motor."

Hopefully, it is appreciated that a lens does nothing to a person. On the contrary, a person can do much with a lens. What, then, does a lens do? And what, in reality, does a person do with lenses placed in front of a pair of eyes? Consideration must be given to the visual process, its mechanisms and its biomechanical requirements to answer these questions. What better way to begin this discussion than with the consideration of the eye? What role does the eye (eyes) play in the visual process?

Gordon Walls, Ph.D., physiologist, once said, "Vision is the product of a very simple eye and a most complex brain." This statement should not be taken too literally as Walls wanted to make people realize there was more to an understanding of vision than a simple knowledge of the eye. Indeed, it is questionable that the eye is simple. Such a statement is much easier for the student of vision to accept as compared to one who makes a study of the eye his life-long endeavor. Nevertheless, no one could disagree with a statement that an eyeball has no vision. Yet, the process of vision depends on the existence of an eyeball and, in the human being at least, on the existence of a pair of eyeballs under ordinary conditions.

In *Notes on a Dynamic Theory of Vision*,[1] referring to earlier discussed static concepts of vision, Harmon wrote,

The visual theories referred to earlier would seem to imply that the eye and its immediately related structures are endowed with all the characteristics necessary to determine the properties, nature and meaning of situations, objects and forms lying in visual space. This is not borne out by the data on which those theories are constructed.

Close examination of standard ophthalmological and other visual literature shows that the existence of these characteristics of the 'eye' are only assumed. Existing evidence supports no other characteristics inherent in the optical, retinal and immediately connected neural mechanisms of the eye than the so-called 'light sense.'

...we concluded that the only 'sense' inherent in the eye itself was probably the 'light sense.' In view of this, the only logical conclusion which can be reached is that the contribution of the optical and retinal mechanisms to visual perception and visual performance is some configuration of neural signals implying the light density pattern of apparent visual space.

The optical and retinal functions of the eye serve the organism as a light distribution or light gradient detector, with their individual and combined operations functioning to define differences in the distribution of light energy, or define light gradient steps in different areas of the visual field, with sufficient acuteness in different segments of the visual field to meet the needs of the organism in adjusting to its external surround.[1]

In other words, the "simple" eye is a composite of two prime mechanisms, (1) the optical mechanism, and (2) the retinal mechanism. The optical mechanism is a superbly designed adjustable convex lens system resplendent with such necessary characteristics as spherical aberration, coma and chromatic aberration. Unfortunately, the word aberration used to describe these characteristics tends to suggest these are undesirables. Perhaps this is so in a discussion of camera optics, but this is definitely not valid in any consideration of the function of the eye.

The retinal mechanism is a complex neural network specifically designed to receive and respond to light distribution. The eye, as a structure, is designed to receive, accept and distribute light over the neural network referred to as the retina. And with this, in reality, begins the elaborate process of vision. You should recall the definition of vision: *the deriving of meaning and directing of action as a product of processing information triggered by a selected band of radiant energy (light).*

Referring back to an earlier statement that a lens does nothing to a person but a person may do much with a lens, it can be said that a lens does something to an eye. Related to the optical mechanism of the eye, any lens placed in front of an eye is added to and becomes a part of the eye's convex lens system. The resultant of this addition to the optical mechanism in turn influences (affects) the retinal mechanism. The light distribution over the retina is altered. The neural signals initiated at the retinal level by the light distribution represent the light-related input from which vision ultimately emerges. Thus, the imposition of a lens in front of an eye results in a change in input. Conveying information to be processed, these neural signals represent only one aspect of information totally utilized in processing centers from which vision emerges. As a derivative of this insight, Skeffington pointed out (as noted earlier) that the value of a lens is that it changes the orders to the system.

The foregoing is an over-simplified description of the initiating of the visual process. It is not a description of the process itself. Prior to the deriving of meaning and directing of action, the processing of information involves the fulfillment of certain fundamental commitments on the part of the organism once action is triggered by the "light sense."

It has long been recognized that at least 20% of the retinal fibers lead to the posturing mechanisms of the body rather than to the higher centers. The first order commitment required of the body as a product of information processing is to come to a balance with gravity desirably with a minimum amount of effort expended. In addition to numerous other dynamic mechanisms of posture involved, this activity embodies the mechanisms of convergence and accommodation. Thus emerges the body's appreciation of "where it is." Not until these two commitments have been realized can the organism proceed to the higher order of information processing and "manipulate the task" and derive "what it is"—the ultimate deriving of meaning and directing of action or the emergent—which is vision. Task manipulation, the last order activity, involves what Skeffington referred to as "centering and identification." The efficiency and adequacy of the third order of information processing depends on the ease with which the initial two commitments are fulfilled. Hence, the statement associated with both desirably coming to balance with minimum amount of effort (energy) expended so that maximum energy is available for task manipulation. The more effort required in satisfying the initial commitments of balance, the less efficient the deriving of meaning and directing of action, which is stress inducing and ultimately requires the organism to "grow along a line of stress to reduce stress." This is identified, then, as a dysfunction in the visual process. Perhaps one of the most startling aspects is that only 200 milliseconds are available for the total neurological process triggered by the "light sense." If the information is not processed within this time, it must be processed again or ignored, which is ineffective and inefficient.

Information processing is experienced as movements, both overt and covert. These movement patterns are described as orientation and localization. Orientation describes the body's coming to balance with gravity and with the task. This involves the posturing mechanisms associated with these activities. On the other hand, localization is a derivative of the body's coming to balance on the task and manipulating the task. It should be noted that the commitment of coming to balance with the task demand is common to both orientation and localization. In terms of balancing mechanisms, orientation involves the lower back muscles, localization involves the upper back and neck musculature.

K. Wells writes, "Probably the only time the human body is not adjusting itself in response to gravitational force is when it is in a position of repose, either lying down or reclining with all its parts completely supported. Either consciously or unconsciously, man spends most of his waking hours adjusting his position in order to resist the pull of gravity upon his body."[2] In other words, unless the body is "in repose," as Wells states, the body is always in balance. It is inappropriate to describe the non-reposed body as being out of balance. How the body is in balance is the critical factor. Balance, at any given moment, describes the forces derived from supportive musculature of the body that play on the body from which is derived a center of gravity. Balance is a dynamic process and this center of gravity shifts with every movement. The center may shift up or down, side-to-side, and/or forward and backward, depending on the action of the forces.

Harmon's electromyographic studies revealed conclusively how the imposition of lenses influences orientation and localization. Fundamentally, the addition of lenses to the convex optical system changes the light distribution on the retina. This alters how one comes to balance with gravity and it influences task manipulation. The essential change is reflected in the degree of muscular tonicity. For example, addition of plus lens power reduces supportive musculature tonicity. Reduction of plus, or increasing minus lens power, increases the tonicity. Addition of excessive amounts of plus creates an alarmingly high degree of hypo-tonicity that could lead literally to atrophy, whereas inadequate plus, permitting a state of hyper-tonicity, could result in various other forms of maladaptation as the organism would grow along a line of stress in order to reduce stress.

Increased tonicity of lower back musculature results in a shift of the center of gravity forward of the norm. Hypo-tonicity permits a shift of the gravitational center in the reversed direction. As a product of his insight and appreciation of body adaptation, Harmon could inspect postural status and, from this, derive the refractive status. As an example, the myope is one within whom the center of gravity has shifted forward and, as a total postural result of adaptation, is seen as one "who leads with his chin." The adverse hyperope is exactly opposite, "leading with his forehead." In the final analysis and with complete insight into these processes, it can be demonstrated that all ocular defects are, in reality, reflections of postural alterations viewed optometrically. This results in the adjustments and adaptations of postural mechanisms required to come to balance with gravity as well as the task demands of life.

Recognizing the Skeffington statement—the value of a lens is that it changes the orders to the system—it can be appreciated that the change in orders is directed to the posturing mechanism of the body, not higher order mechanisms. Thus, "a lens does nothing to a person" save altering light distribution, but "a person may do much with a lens."

The value and purpose of the stress-relieving lens relates to the potential and availability of alteration of the musculature involved in balancing mechanisms. This is exactly what the stresspoint retinoscope reveals, i.e., what lens formula can be utilized, and utilizing the data of the analytical examination and denoting the value of such a lens to the individual based on the degree of embeddedness. This is in contrast to the value and/or need of compensatory lenses to an individual.

When an individual has made adaptation within his postural mechanisms to the extent that the optometric examination reveals an ocular defect such as myopia, adverse hyperopia and/or astigmatism, it should be understood that the identifiable ocular defect is the end result and it is revealed in the inner optics of the eye. These limitations in visual acuity may be detrimental and/or restrictive. Compensatory lenses may be required to enable adequate visual acuity for adequate visual performance. Contrary to prior inappropriate use of terminology, such lenses are not correcting lenses. They correct nothing. Such lenses, if utilized properly, do not alter nor influence the postural mechanisms. However, such lenses alter the light distribution on the retina as a result of being added to the optical mechanism of the eye. The retinal signals (input) are affected by altering the light distribution. There is, in the language of the electronic engineer, a reduction in noise level and an increase in information quality.

It would appear that the movement pattern activities of orientation and localization could involve, to a degree, one without the other. This is a built-in protective function and it describes the range (or latitude) of freedom. Recall that orientation is a description of the refractive status of the body and directly reflects the status of the lower back posturing musculature.

Localization directly involves the upper back and neck musculature and describes spatial computing status. The latter refers to one who sees objects coincident with the emanating energy force, or closer than or farther away than that force. It also relates to spatial constancy and consistency. The influence of such behavior is detectable in the postural adjustments within the scapula. For example, flat scapulae are indicative of a tendency to see objects nearer in space as compared to reality, which Harmon termed esophoric performance. Exophoric performance describes the opposite status with the scapulae winging outward.

The use of such optometric terms to describe these behavioral adaptations should not be confused with, nor implied to be equivalent to, similar terms that describe specific measurements revealed from standard optometric examination procedures.

Further exploration of involved musculature associated with visual performance suggests that against-the-rule astigmatism is a reflection of orientation musculature whereas with-the-rule astigmatism is related to localization. Oblique astigmatism is a resultant of involvement of the total musculature.

With the understanding that the terms binocular and monocular are used to describe conditions of input, the following observations can be cited and demonstrated clinically on a two-eyed individual:

1. Orientation is directly altered by
   a. Binocular spheres and
   b. Monocular prism or binocular yoked prism
2. Localization is directly altered by
   a. Monocular spheres and
   b. Binocular base-out or base-in prism

The foregoing is seen easily with the aid of a retinoscope in addition to direct observation of the convergence mechanism. A retinoscope will reveal discernible changes in the accommodative mechanism.

For example, the retinoscope will reveal motion change with the imposition of binocular spheres while the subject is fixating a given object equivalent to the lens value added to the optical mechanism. Assuming the retinoscope initially reveals neutrality, addition of binocular plus results in "against" motion and thus, no changes in the crystalline lens convexity. On the other hand, the placement of a sphere before one eye results in a crystalline change (as well as convergence change) under monocular conditions with the same initial retinoscopic observation so that the reflex seen by retinoscopy equals that seen prior to the placement of the lens.

Likewise, placement before the eyes of binocular base-out or base-in prism will reveal a resulting change in the accommodation mechanism and convergence mechanism. Finally, retinoscopy reveals no change in the mechanisms of accommodation or convergence, if either monocular prism or binocular yoked prism (bases-up, -down, -right or -left) is placed before the subject under the same conditions. The only change noted is in the direction of eyes, the eyes turning specifically in the direction of the prism apex.

Hopefully, this chapter will provide insight, understanding, appreciation and substance to preceding chapters, and set the stage for later chapters.

References
1. Harmon DB. Notes on a dynamic theory of vision. Austin, Texas: Privately published, 1958:60-65.
2. Wells K. Kinesiology. Philadelphia: W. B. Saunders, 1960:339.

CHAPTER 7
Myopia: The Behavioral View

Sir W. Stewart Duke-Elder wrote: "The fibers from the retina end in two masses of gray matter: the lateral geniculate body, which is phylogenetically part of the optic thalamus, and the superior colliculus, which is part of the mid-brain.... The visual fibers (in man) find a relay station in the lateral geniculate body.... Eighty percent of the retinal fibers find their way here.... The retinal fibers which run to the superior colliculus, however, are undoubtedly the most primitive phylogenetically...and in man they are associated with the primitive photostatic (light and posture) rather than the higher sensory functions of vision."[1]

The key to the understanding (and ultimate application) of the behavioral concept of vision and the visual process (and all of its ramifications) is an appreciation of the significance of these other 20% of retinal fibers. These fibers lead to lower centers and "are associated with the primitive photostatic" functions of the visual process.

Conventional wisdom has all but ignored this reality. Notions (other than the behavioral) from which clinical care directives have emerged give no consideration at all to this extremely important aspect of the visual process. This limited insight results in a restricted point of view, one that minimizes the quality of vision care and limits the role of the optometrist as well as the profession of optometry itself.

Reference was made in Chapter 6 to the retinal fibers associated with the photostatic functions. It was noted that all ocular defects are reflections of postural alterations and adaptations. The term ocular defect(s) is used deliberately to connote any optometrically viewed deviation from the expectations of the unimpaired visual process. More specifically, refractive status and extraocular muscle status, i.e., phorias (both horizontal and vertical) and strabismus, are optometrically viewed reflections of postural involvement; they relate to the functions of orientation and localization.

Myopia is the most common example of an ocular defect, as defined above. When myopia is identified, extensive consideration should be given to the behavioral optometric rationale and clinical approach. Myopia is generally viewed as a condition of the visual system. The how and why of myopia and the clinical approach to a patient with myopia are variants of the optometrist's point of view and/or concept.

Myopia is defined and described in many ways—etiologically, structurally, functionally, and operationally. The definition varies according to the definer's concept of vision. The definition is colored frequently by assumptions that are stated as facts. When this is the case, such a definition can be dangerous for it may delimit the user in his thinking and clinical application.

An excellent example is the unfortunate standard definition of myopia given to first-year optometry students, i.e., Myopia: "That condition wherein rays of light focus in front of the retina." Such a definition implies structural fault of an eye; it delimits the clinical approach. Actually, this definition, itself, is contrary to the realities of the beautiful optical system of the eye, as described in Chapter 6.

The best and safest definition is one that is free of assumptions and implications. This is best labeled an operational definition or description.

A. M. Skeffington provides an excellent operational definition of myopia, when he states that myopia is that condition in which visual acuity is less than standard but restored to standard with concave lenses.

In Chapter 4, the behavioral concept of the etiology of vision dysfunction was described. That chapter stated that vision dysfunction results either from interference in the developing process of vision, i.e., vision development problems, and/or from interference in the developed process, i.e., stress-induced visual problems. (By far, the latter is the most common seen clinically.) Although myopia may result as a product of thwarting development, it is extremely rare. It is extreme when revealed, and, usually, it has existed since before age 4.

Most myopia occurs in response to stress induced by the biologically unacceptable, visually compulsive, near-centered task performed by the individual. In reality, the stress-induced visual problem is the condition, and the myopia is the mode of adaptation. Recall that there are two major routes of adaptation in response to stress: (1) myopia, and (2) syndrome of reduced visual efficiency. The majority of people develop the latter. It should be noted here (with discussion held until later) that there is an alternative to myopia which some people experience as a temporary or permanent adaptation. This is divergent strabismus.

Clinically, myopia is seen both as a primary adaptation and a secondary response. By definition, primary myopia is that which emerges in the visual process as an initial response to the imposed stress. This is the myopia that occurs in the early school years. However, clinicians are well aware of myopia occurring in high school years, college years, and even later. This is secondary myopia. With the evidence at hand and insightful differential diagnosis, it is evident that secondary myopia occurs as a secondary response to additional stress; in actuality, the patient was affected earlier by a syndrome of reduced visual efficiency.

Contrary to a person who is affected by the syndrome of reduced efficiency, myopia is a means to preserve an individual's cultural efficiency by sacrificing distance visual acuity. That is, the myopia gives up at farpoint in order to perform at near; whereas the more common adaptation is seen in a patient who maintains standard visual acuity but gives up efficiency instead of intellectual capability.

In reality, it can be expected that myopes are better achievers by sixth grade in an average classroom. One could conclude, then, that myopia is a rather intelligent adaptation; that is, if one must have a visual disability. However, no rationalization should dignify or justify the development of a vision condition if it can be prevented or altered. If one is myopic, the fact remains that there is a restriction in the ability to see and appropriate vision care is required. This is but another example of the importance of the concept of vision. After all, it is the concept that dictates what is appropriate vision care. Appropriate vision care, according to the conventional point of view, is the prescription of concave lenses. This provides standard visual acuity at farpoint, generally, for constant wear without consideration of comfort, let alone further myopic progression. In fact, the general underlying implication is: "Here's a pair of glasses you can see with; come back and get stronger glasses when you get worse." And, indeed, this is exactly what many people still do because they do not know any better.

On the other hand, the behavioral concept requires that the optometrist direct his attention and professional expertise to (1) the prevention of visual problems, and (2) the control, maintenance, and improvement of visual performance. As stated earlier, myopia, simply, is viewed as one mode of adaptation within the visual process—not as a separate entity.

Appropriate vision care will be determined by the desires and needs of the patient as evidenced from the diagnostic interpretation of data collected by the optometrist. If a vision condition exists, the data will reveal it. Additionally, the data will reveal the status of adaptation and the potential benefits of lenses and/or formalized visual training. Obviously, if the patient is myopic, the data will reveal what concave lenses are required to achieve standard distance or near visual acuity. (When reference is made to concave lenses, this refers to regular ophthalmic lenses or contact lenses.)

However, the optometrist when confronted with a patient showing signs of myopia should consider several questions. They include the following: Does the patient need standard visual acuity? Is it in the patient's best interest to provide such concave lenses? If required, how should and when should the patient use such concave lenses? Can anything be recommended to prevent further myopic progression? How can visual performance be controlled and maintained? Can the condition be altered or reversed? If so, how and with what?

Contrary to conventional wisdom, the behavioral approach recognizes that the degree of myopia varies with the viewing distance. The optical concept of vision implies that myopia is myopia is myopia—the implication being that myopia is a defect of the eyeball(s) and standard measurement of the degree of myopia is at farpoint. The behavioral optometrist appreciates that (1) myopia is NOT a defect of an eyeball, and (2) when discussing a patient as being myopic, it must be described as myopia at what distance.

As stated above, it is important to remember that myopia varies with viewing distance. Recalling Skeffington's operational definition, myopia cannot exist if one has standard visual acuity. When myopia initially emerges as the mode of adaptation, visual acuity will be substandard at farpoint, but visual acuity is standard at nearpoint. Visual acuity at farpoint will be restored to standard with concave lenses

In this example, it would be proper to state that the patient is myopic at farpoint, but not at near. As it progresses, myopia, ultimately, is revealed at nearpoint, but it is always less than at farpoint. The patient may require one dioptric value for standard acuity at farpoint, but less at near.

This author has never seen the reverse, and he finds it totally inconceivable that the reverse could exist. It can never be in the best interest of any patient with myopia to prescribe—based on a distance measurement of myopia—a single pair of concave lenses to be worn constantly. One should understand that concave lenses, which provide standard visual acuity at farpoint, must represent significantly greater compensation than that required at near. In other words, use of such lenses at near is overcompensation and no different from prescribing excessive minus lenses at farpoint.

Undoubtedly, one of the major reasons that the degree of myopia continues to progress is due to the use of excessive minus at near. This causes continued stress and it requires continued maladaptation. If never given any concave lenses, the chances are great that the patient probably will create from 2.50 to 3.00 diopters of myopia as measured at far with no myopia at near.

The behavioral approach views myopia as an optometric reflection of the total person that delimits visual performance. It is a reflection of postural alteration and adaptation. Specifically, the optometric measurements reveal the end result seen in the inner optics of the eyes, an excessive convex lens system.

Restoring standard distance visual acuity by applying concave lenses is simply the algebraic product of reducing the convexity of the system. This permits a more appropriate light density gradient distribution on the retina and it results in better quality information as input. However, the imposition of concave lenses does not alter the myopia because the myopia is IN the person; it is now a physical component of the body.

A review of Chapter 6 will demonstrate that myopia is a reflection of body postural change resulting in the center of gravity moving forward of the norm. Also, a review will reveal the significant impact on the body posturing muscles as the result of imposing convex and concave lenses in front of the eyes.

The general principle is that convex lenses reduce tonicity and concave lenses increase tonicity. An appreciation of these principles is the foundation to an understanding of the behavioral use of lenses.

As stated above, the use of minus lenses for near, when not required for standard acuity, results in increased myopia. Minus lenses increase the tonicity of the posturing muscles of the body. This increase results in a shifting of the center of gravity forward of the norm—hence, increased myopia.

Perhaps now it is understood why this author stated earlier in this chapter that the key to understanding the behavioral concept of vision and the visual process (and all its ramifications) is an appreciation of the significance of the 20% of retinal fibers which lead to lower centers and "are associated with the primitive photostatic" functions of the visual process.

The Myope: Needs, Wants, and Desires

The knowledge, experience, and services of an optometrist offering a behavioral approach are an advantage to an individual seeking vision care. Such an assessment has special relevance to considerations in myopia.

Fundamentally, a behavioral approach has more to offer any patient than an approach using, what shall be labeled the conventional-wisdom. As has been discussed in this book, an understanding of the *dynamic functional concept of vision* of a behavioral approach provides the opportunity to satisfy more effectively the needs, wants, and desires of individuals seeking vision care.

The principal advantage of treatment by an optometrist with a behavioral orientation is that, by virtue of basic education and training, the optometrist has insight to, as well as an appreciation of, conventional-wisdom approaches to vision care. Yet, this optometrist also has an extended base of knowledge to include the more elaborate and exciting aspects of the behavioral aspects of optometric care. Contrary to what some believe, the conventional-wisdom approach and the behavioral approach are not at opposite ends of a horizontal scale. Rather, it is best shown as a vertical continuum. In other words, the behavioral approach has emerged as a product of continuous development; and the an optometrist with a behavioral orientation is one whose education has been expanded beyond the base of knowledge, also known as conventional-wisdom. The behaviorally oriented optometrist, then, includes the knowledge, understanding, and insight of the implications and limitations of conventional-wisdom.

An optometrist limited to the conventional wisdom aspects of optometry cannot appreciate the realities and applications of the dynamic functional concept of vision because of never having been exposed to the concept. This author has never known an optometrist to understand or develop insights of the *behavioral concept* and, then choose to practice within the confines imposed by conventional-wisdom optometry.

The optometrist with a behavioral approach has a greater opportunity to satisfy the needs, wants and desires of the patient more effectively, if these needs, wants and desires are reasonable. But, what is reasonable?

Several questions were asked earlier in this chapter, which should be considered by the optometrist when treating a patient showing signs of myopia. It should be emphasized that these are probably questions that are asked also by patients, if not verbally, then, mentally. In other words, patients are as interested as the practitioner to learn and define their needs, wants and desires. For the reader's review, the questions are as follows:

Does the patient need standard visual acuity?

Is it in the patient's best interest to provide concave lenses?

If required, how should and when should the patient use concave lenses?

Can anything be recommended to prevent further myopic progression?

How can visual performance be controlled and maintained?

Can the condition be altered or reversed? If so, how and with what?

These questions are unique in that they are relevant only to the behavioral approach to optometric care. However, the answers to such questions will vary and they will be influenced by the thinking and understanding of the optometrist providing the vision care.

After 32 years of practice, this author cannot recall one patient who wanted to become more myopic. Of course, it is doubtful that any myopic patient desires to be myopic, but this may not be a reasonable expectation.

Case Example

Miss EY, age 25, was seen by this author on April 8, 1981 for her initial optometric diagnostic examination and evaluation. She was a writer for a prominent national magazine. Her prescription, provided two years earlier by another examiner was OD -.75 sphere, OS -0.25 -0.50 x 65.

She first became aware of difficulty seeing at a distance, six years earlier, when she was in college. She was then given compensatory lenses for the first time. The glasses from two years ago were just her second pair. At the time of examination, she used the glasses selectively for distance. She was never told to avoid use of the glasses for near, but she discovered, herself, it was more comfortable to do without the lenses whenever possible. However, the patient felt that she needed "stronger glasses" because she did not see adequately when using the glasses. The only additional symptom admitted was an awareness of "tired eyes" when reading. Also, the patient said she was satisfied with her level of visual efficiency.

The "eye health screening" revealed the eyes and adnexa to be free from pathology and abnormality.

The data gathered from the optometric examination was as follows:

Unaided visual acuity at far: OD 20/50, OS 20/33, OU 20/29

Unaided visual acuity at near: OD, OS, and OU 20/20

Cover test: ortho far and near

Convergence nearpoint: 2 inches, left eye deviating out and diplopia reported; recovery at 12 inches

Ocular motility: pursuit movements were full and unrestricted but jerky; fixations were accurate

Telebinocular DB series: The complete battery was done. Significant observations were, (1) suppressions were revealed, and (2) DB3 (signboards) was improved with occlusion of left eye

Wirt stereo: #9

The Analytical Examination

#3 (distance habitual phoria)--½ eso   #13A (near habitual phoria)--3 exo

#4 (retinoscopy)   OD -0.25 -0.25 x 55
                         OS +.50 -0.25 x 90

#5 (retinoscopy at 20 inches)   OD +1.25 -0.25 x 55
                                 OS +2.00 -0.25 x 90

#7 (subjective)--OU -0.75 sphere

#8 (phoria through #7)--½ eso
   (Control at far #7)

#9 (base out blur)--X

#10 (base out break/recovery)--12/3

#11 (base in break/recovery)--7/2

#13B (near phoria through #7)--3 exo

#14A (unfused cross cylinder)--OU +0.75

#15A (phoria through #14A)--7 exo

#14B (fused cross cylinder)--OU +0.50

#15B (phoria through #14B)--5 exo
     (Control at near OU Plano)

#16A (base our blur)--X   #16B (base out break/recovery)--9/2

#17A (base in blur)--X   #17B (base in break/recovery)--13/9

#19--4.50 (amplitude of accommodation)

#20-- -3.75 (minus lens to blur out)

#21--+2.75 (plus lens to blur out)

Stresspoint Retinoscope: OU +0.50 provided best balance

ALTERNATIVES OF CARE

After an analysis and an evaluation of the optometric data, as well as a consideration of the questions already stated previously in this chapter, the patient was provided three alternative optometric care programs. By providing her with three alternative programs, the patient was given the opportunity to select the one that would satisfy her needs, wants and desires. The alternatives were as follows:

1. Conventional Care: provide the presently indicated compensatory lenses, permitting better visual acuity as needed; continue to use the glasses as in the past; that is, selectively for distance and not for near. This would require changing the left lens only.

2. Behavioral Care: provide appropriate counter-stress lenses in single vision form to be used for all near-centered activity. The use of such lenses will reduce the current stress, controlling and protecting against additional adverse adaptation of myopia; myopia status may be reversed; expect increase in comfort. Do not modify compensatory lenses yet, and continue to use the old glasses selectively and minimally as before. Return in three months for a reevaluation progress case study.

3. Visual Training: for maximum visual efficiency as well as possibility of myopia reduction and/or elimination with resultant improvement in distance-seeing ability. Six - eight months predicted.

With an understanding of the potential benefits of each alternative and given an opportunity to choose among the three alternatives, the patient selected the second alternative. Apparently, the potential benefits to be derived from this alternative were consistent with what she determined her needs, wants and desires to be.

It should be noted that the optometrist with a behavioral approach does not determine and dictate a program of optometric care to the patient. Rather, the optometrist analyzes and evaluates the data collected from the optometric examination. Then, alternative programs of care are made available to the patient. These alternatives always include the only approach associated with and provided by conventional wisdom clinicians. This approach preserves patients' abilities to select the level of care that best answers their needs, wants and desires. (As an aside, it is extremely interesting that only about 10% of the patient population, provided the choices of a behavioral approach, select conventional-wisdom care, when supplied with these alternatives of vision care.)

Care Provided

Having selected alternative number two, the prescription provided was OU +0.50 spheres—equivalent to the stresspoint retinoscope finding. The lenses were to be used for all visually near-centered activities.

EY returned for her progress case study in September, when she reported that she used the stress-relieving lenses consistently for all near work. She reported no discomfort. She no longer had "tired eyes" and was not aware of any additional limitation in distance seeing. Recall that she had used the compensatory lenses selectively for distance when needed; this included driving, television, movies, etc. Since using the new lenses for near, she felt the need for the compensatory lenses only when driving; otherwise, she was not aware of any distance-seeing restrictions.

Without providing the data of the entire reevaluation examination, the following should be known:

Unaided visual acuity at far: OD 20/29, OS 20/25, OU 20/22

#13A (near habitual phoria) (Plano)--1 exo

#7 (subjective)--OU -0.25 sph.

#13B (near phoria with OU +0.50)--3 exo

#16B (near base out break/recovery with near Rx)--18/6

#17B (near base in break/recovery with near Rx)--21/6

Stresspoint Retinoscope: OU +0.50 provided best balance

As predicted, there was an obvious change in visual function and performance. Recognizing she was still "in process" of change, EY was instructed to continue as before; that is, to use the counter-stress lenses for all near work and the old distance lenses only when absolutely necessary. Since the compensatory lenses were used so minimally, no change was made in the prescription. She was programmed to return in six months for the next reevaluation examination.

EY was seen in March 1982 for this progress case study. Again, she reported no discomfort associated with near-centered demands and she was most satisfied with her level of efficiency. She was not aware of any significant limitation in distance seeing with the exception of some night driving; and she used her compensatory lenses only when needed. The significant observations of this office visit were as follows:

Unaided visual acuity at far: OD and OS 20/22, OU 20/20

#7 (subjective) OU Plano

Stresspoint Retinoscope: OU +0.50 provided best balance

She was instructed to continue the use of the plus lenses for near and, as before, minimal, if any, use of the compensatory lenses. She was programmed to be seen for an annual complete reevaluation examination in one year.

The case of EY is a common one in optometric offices. However, the approach is one unique to the office providing a behavioral approach to optometric care.

The collection of data, its analysis, and its evaluation were completed within the framework of the behavioral approach. Initially, the data revealed that her myopia was a secondary adaptation to a previously existing stress-induced dysfunction associated with reduced visual efficiency. Visual behavior was partially embedded.

Experience demonstrates that secondary myopia is more alterable than primary myopia. By definition, myopia that results as a primary adaptation to the stress of near-centered demands is labeled "primary myopia." Secondary myopia arises as a later adaptation and as a product of additional stress imposed by the demands of the environment. This occurs frequently after elementary school years and more commonly in high school and/or college years. An individual with secondary myopia can suffer from reduced visual efficiency without even being aware of it. The incidence of primary myopia is more common, however.

Myopia Classifications

Any discussion of myopia must consider the numerous classifications, which relate to clinical directives and patient approaches. The etiological classification of primary and secondary myopia associated with stress-induced visual dysfunction is just one example. Operationally, there is another and more pragmatic classification.

Myopes fall into three operational categories. These are as follows:

1. The myope who has never had compensatory lenses for distance
2. The myope who has compensatory lenses but uses such lenses selectively for distance
3. The myope who has compensatory lenses and uses such lenses constantly for distance (and possibly always)

The significance of these classifications is that they relate both to the needs, wants and desires of an individual, as well as the ultimate optometric recommendations.

Visual Training

Although these chapters deliberately have avoided discussion of formalized visual training, the author is compelled to offer some comments on visual training, this operational classification, and the desires of many myopic patients to improve their distance seeing.

In terms of acceptability as a patient for visual training with the goal of improvement in distance seeing (and assuming the patient is old enough to be motivated personally to do so, i.e., not a parent decision), the prognosis for improvement and altered behavior is excellent for the myope who has never had compensatory lenses. Prognosis is good also for the myope who uses compensatory lenses selectively. If nothing else, this myope probably will improve his ability to see at a distance for the time he does not use glasses. It may be discovered also that the selective need for such lenses is reduced.

However, the prognosis is poor for the myope who uses glasses constantly. Usually, such a patient is not acceptable in the author's office for visual training.

Guidelines for Myopia Care

Recall the degree of myopia is a function of the viewing distance, and, operationally, the degree of myopia is determined by the amount of concave lens power required to restore standard visual acuity. Consequently, general guidelines for the behavioral approach to myopia can be established. These guidelines, which answer the fundamental questions raised previously, are as follows:

1. Never prescribe compensatory lens power greater than that required for standard visual acuity.
2. Prescribe only that degree of compensatory lens power required to meet the needs of the patient.
3. Never insist that a selective user of compensatory lenses use such lenses constantly.
4. Never insist that a myope who has never had compensatory lenses use such lenses unless his needs require it, and then, if so, suggest that the patient always be selective in such use.
5. Always identify the degree of myopia, if any, at nearpoint, and offer the appropriate opportunity to use such lenses or other identified stress-relieving lenses for near in order to protect, control, and maintain visual behavior.
6. Always analyze and evaluate the total collection of optometric data so as to know the status of adaptation (i.e., degree of embeddedness) and to apprise the patient of the potential benefits derived from the Behavioral Concept.

The determination of the degree of myopia at farpoint is the #7 finding. The degree of minus lens compensation prescribed for distance, if any, is based on professional judgment, utilizing the guideline criteria listed above. On the other hand, the determination of the degree of myopia at near is determined by the minimum amount of concave lens power required for standard visual acuity at the patient's nearpoint, using the reduced Snellen acuity chart. The specific lens power prescribed for near, however, in the author's office, is the stresspoint retinoscope finding. The benefits to be gained by the patient are determined by the complete case analysis and evaluation.

Reference
1. Duke-Elder, WS. Textbook of ophthalmology, Vol. I. St. Louis: C. V. Mosby: 247-248.

CHAPTER 8
What Power Hath A Lens?

The theme of these chapters is that human behavior can be altered as a product of the benefits derived from the power of lenses.

Unfortunately, a behavioral approach to optometry is equated frequently with optometric visual training. The terms are used inappropriately and interchangeably as though they are one and the same. They are not.

In fact, visual training emerged from an understanding and appreciation of the utilization of lenses. This, in turn, emerges from an understanding and appreciation of the *Dynamic Functional Concept of Vision—the Behavioral Aspects of Optometry.* Unquestionably, visual training represents the glamour of optometry. But, the excitement of optometry evolves from the benefits experienced by the patient through the utilization of lenses.

The following case is presented to illustrate the excitement that is optometry. It shows the benefits received by a patient from a simple application of lenses. This case best exemplifies the insight derived from the behavioral concept.

A Case Report

Patient SF, a young man, age 21, was examined by the author in June, after he had just completed the first semester of his junior year at a small state college. Up to that time he had never had any program of vision care. Although he was last examined by a non-optometric examiner about three years earlier, no diagnosis or recommendations were made.

He reported seeing clearly, but he experienced tired and burning eyes after studying. He had always been a poor student, and he had had spelling and handwriting problems. Significantly, his early history revealed that he had motor coordination difficulties and problems in learning to read well.

In earlier years, he had undergone special educational testing outside school; one series of tests suggested the possibility of visual dysfunction. However, subsequent professional examination did not identify any visual problem. (This is an excellent example of what some call "over-referral," but which, in reality, is "under-examination.")

SF also reported his reading as slow and tedious; he had to reread for comprehension. He preferred learning auditorially instead of reading and/or studying.

The investigation of eye health status revealed the eyes and adnexa as free of pathology and abnormality. The data gathered from the optometric examination were as follows:

Unaided visual acuity at far and near: OD, OS and OU 20/20

Cover test: ortho at far; exophoria and right hyperphoria at near

Convergence nearpoint: 8 inches, right eye deviating out and diplopia reported; recovery at 10 inches

Ocular motility: pursuit movements were full and unrestricted but very poor; fixations were poor

Preferred eye was left but he was right-handed

Head position: tilted left, turned right; forced head tilt to right induced diplopia

Visual Abilities (Telebinocular, DB Series):

> DB10 (pig and dog): both present with suppression
> DB8 (line and ball): right hyper with suppression
> DB4K (3 balls): 2 balls vertically fused
> DB6D (stereopsis): #12
> DB3 and DB2 (signboards): 20/17
> DB9 (far) (arrow and numbers): #8
> DB9 (near) (arrow and numbers): #4
> DB5K (3 balls at near): 2 balls vertically fused

WIRT stereo: #9

The Analytical Sequence:

#3 (habitual distance phoria)--4 eso   #13A (habitual near phoria)--4 exo

#4 (retinoscopy)　　　　　　　OD +0.50 -0.75 x 90
　　　　　　　　　　　　　　　OS +0.25 -0.50 x 80

#5 (retinoscopy at 20 inches)　OD +2.00 -0.75 x 95
　　　　　　　　　　　　　　　OS +1.50 -0.50 x 80

#7 (subjective)　　　　　　　　OD +0.25 sphere
　　　　　　　　　　　　　　　OS Plano

#8 (phoria through #7)--4 eso
　(Control at far: OU Plano)

#9 (base out blur)--X   #10 (base out break/recovery)--10/no recovery, vertical separation

#11 (base in break/recovery)--6/no recovery, vertical separation

#12 (distance vertical phoria)--3 right hyper

#13B (near phoria through #7)--4 exo

#14A (unfused cross cylinder)--OU +0.50 sphere

#15A (phoria through #14A)--8 exo

#14B (fused cross cylinder)--Vertical diplopia

#16 through #21: No measures attainable due to vertical diplopia

#18 (vertical phoria at near)--10 right hyper

Stresspoint retinoscope: OU +0.75 sphere provided best balance

Obviously, the data revealed something other than the patient's history suggested.

As the vertical disability revealed itself in the course of the examination (first, the Telebinocular and secondly, the cover test), the examiner was compelled to probe patient history further. Two thoughts prevailed: (1) SF was last examined three years ago; the lack of a diagnosis or recommendation suggested that a vertical disability did not exist then; and (2) there was no reported diplopia of any sort at any time.

Experience suggested that such conditions are associated frequently with some form of back and/or neck problems—usually, transient conditions resulting from a trauma, such as automobile accidents. As such, the patient was questioned further.

Indeed, he was a victim of two automobile accidents. The first was two years ago. The second was less than 10 months ago. He confirmed again that he had no diplopia, but he reported periodic pain at mid-back level. It was concluded, therefore, that the vertical disability was the product of a back trauma to which he had adapted. This would not be considered, then, in the analysis and interpretation of the optometric data related to visual function.

An evaluation of the collected optometric data and information (excluding data related to the back trauma) suggested that SF had a deep-seated vision development problem and a secondary stress-induced dysfunction. The former contributed to and created early problems in learning; it was an example of a learning-related visual problem. The discomfort resulted from the inadequacy of the visual system to respond to required visual demand. It was the famous S. Howard Bartley, who said, "Discomfort arises when visual efficiency is lower than that satisfactory to the organism."[1]

SF was an excellent candidate for visual training. We finally would have the opportunity to develop and restore desirable and adequate visual abilities as well as the freedom to utilize those abilities in order to develop a more efficient and effective visual process.

That is, if conditions were ideal; however, conditions were not ideal. SF was home from college for only a brief period and he could not be available for visual training. Also, he could not be referred to anyone in his college town. Nobody there could provide this type of vision care.

Two other alternatives were available. The first was the conventional approach to which he had been subjected three years earlier. Essentially, this was a "do-nothing" approach because he had 20/20, healthy eyes and no ocular defects. This was no answer and no help. The second alternative was the potential use of counter-stress lenses.

Although the optometric data could not be analyzed in the usual manner as to the status of adaptation in time (i.e., degree of embeddedness), the stresspoint retinoscope revealed an available stress-reducing lens value. When used for all near work, such lenses could be recommended to reduce current stress. This would allow for increased comfort and ability to sustain on a near-centered task.

This was the accepted approach. However, such an approach was not expected to alleviate the dysfunction. (Hopefully, it would permit him to function more effectively and comfortably.) Therefore, he was prescribed OU +0.75 spheres in single vision form to be used for all near-centered activities, and he was programmed for a reevaluation examination in December.

SF returned for his programmed progress case study on December 28th. He said he had used the counter-stress lenses consistently for all near-centered work. He also reported that he was aware of significantly less discomfort and he was able to sustain on his near work for longer periods of time before his eyes tired or burned. Still, he saw clearly at far and near, and no diplopia existed. He also said he had less back pain.

The optometric data follows:

Unaided visual acuity at far and near: OD, OS, OU 20/20

Cover test: ortho at far and near

Convergence nearpoint: 2 inches, right deviating out and diplopia reported; recovery at 7 inches

Ocular motility: pursuit movements were full and fair

The Analytical data:

#3 (habitual distance phoria)--1 ½ eso #13A (habitual near phoria)--2 exo

#4 (retinoscopy) OD +0.50 -0.50 x 90
OS +0.25 -0.50 x 85

#5 (retinoscopy at 20 inches) OD +2.00 -0.50 x 90
OS +1.75 -0.50 x 85

#7 (subjective)--OU +0.50 spheres

#8 (phoria through #7)--½ eso
(Control at far: OU Plano)

#9 (base out blur)--X

#10 (base our break/recovery)--16/2

#11 (base in break/recovery)--8/1

#12 (vertical phoria)--Ortho

#13B (near phoria through #7)--5 exo
(Control at near: OU +0.75 spheres)

#16A (base out blur)--X #16B (base out break/recovery)--11/2

#17A (base in blur)--X #17B (base in break/recovery)--19/16

#18 (vertical phoria)--2 right hyper

Stresspoint retinoscope: OU +0.75 spheres provided best balance

The patient, then, was aware of the benefits, which resulted from use of the lenses for close work. He was more comfortable and he was able to do near-centered activities for longer periods of time. It was incidental to him that the back pain had lessened.

However, the benefits realized by the patient could not match this examiner's excitement as the optometric data was collected. What had happened to the vertical disability? Where had it gone? What power hath a lens? Were the use of lenses and the dissipation of the hyperphoria related?

The patient was instructed to continue use of the lenses as before. He was scheduled to return for another progress case study at the conclusion of the academic year; however, he was again told that visual training still was the ideal approach to his visual problem.

SF was seen for his reevaluation examination the following May. The results follow:

Unaided visual acuity at far and near: OD, OS, OU 20/20

Cover test: ortho at far and near

Convergence nearpoint: 1 inch, left eye deviating out and diplopia reported; recovery at 4 inches

Ocular motility: pursuit movements were full and fair

Preferred eye was right eye (original examination revealed left eye preferred)

The Analytical Sequence:

#3 (habitual distance phoria)--3 eso   #13A (habitual near phoria)--1 exo

#4 (retinoscopy)   OD +0.50 spheres
                          OS +0.25 spheres

#5 (retinoscopy at 20 inches)--OU +0.50 spheres

#7 (subjective)--OU +0.50 spheres

#8 (phoria through #7)--2 eso
    (Control at far: OU Plano)

#9 (base-out blur)--12

#10 (base-out break/recovery)--18/6

#11 (base-in break/recovery)--7/0

#12 (vertical phoria)--Ortho

#13B (near phoria through #7)--2 exo

#14B (fused cross cylinder)--OU +0.75

#15B (phoria through #14B)--2 exo
    (Control at near: OU +0.75 spheres)

#16A (base-out blur)--14   #16B (base out break/recovery)--15/4

#17A (base-in blur)--12   #17B (base-in break/recovery)--20/14

#18 (vertical phoria)--2 right hyper

#20 (positive relative accommodation)-- -3.75

#21 (negative relative accommodation)--+2.00

Telebinocular, DB Series:

> DB8 (line and ball): ortho, no vertical deviancy revealed
> DB4K (3 balls): 4 balls in eso, no vertical deviancy
> DB5K (3 balls at near): 3 balls, no suppression nor vertical deviancy

Stresspoint retinoscope: OU +0.75 spheres provided best balance

As before, SF reported that he used the stress-relieving lenses for all close work. He had no discomfort and he was able to sustain at near activity as long as required. He was free of any back pain, and most importantly, he ended the college year with the best grades he ever had. In fact, he was so excited about his academic performance that he decided to return to college for summer courses so he could graduate the following year. However, that made the still ideal visual training impractical. So, he was instructed to continue using the lenses and to return in one year for his next programmed reevaluation examination.

The patient was thrilled with the results and benefits of his behavioral optometric program of care. The patient felt that these results exceeded what was anticipated as a product of lens power in action. However, the question in his mind was: If he was able to gain so much with lenses alone, what was his potential if an opportunity existed for visual training? The author asked the same question—and a few others. What happened to the hyperphoria? Where did it go? Why did it dissipate? Were the use of the plus spheres and the change in vertical alignment related?

The stresspoint retinoscopic finding suggested that the plus spheres reduced the stress of near-centered demands. There never was any question that lenses alone could not alleviate the visual dysfunction if this was a vision development problem. But, the use of such lenses could permit one to function more effectively with present level of abilities; this was the result.

This author's rationale for what took place physiologically (and exceeded the benefits initially anticipated) is as follows:
As mentioned earlier, it is not unusual to find a transient effect on ocular-motor status following back trauma related to auto accidents. Frequently, this is seen as hyperphoria, and sometimes it manifests itself as hypertropia with diplopia. The orthopedist refers to this back injury as whiplash. It was not unreasonable, then, to assume that SF's data was so related. Perhaps the condition remained since the more recent accident, which was about 10 months earlier than the initial optometric examination. Contrary to the perseverance of SF's vertical disability, the author's experience suggests that the restoration of normal status is more rapid—usually within two to three months of the accident. Nevertheless, SF revealed the

perseveration of the vertical disability. This could have been the product of a compounding back injury and resulting hyper-tonicities caused by two accidents a little more than a year apart and to which he had maladapted functionally.

The reader should recall that an established fundamental insight associated with the behavioral concept is an appreciation of the significance of the 20% of retinal fibers that lead to lower centers associated with primitive photostatic functions of the visual process. These are the fibers that provide the essential signals of the body coming to balance with gravity and the task at hand. The reader should also recall that non-compensatory lenses' primary influences are on the tonic state of the supporting musculature of the back. Convex lenses reduce tonicity; concave lenses induce tonicity.

The only variable in SF's life from the author's initial examination to completion of both progress case studies was the utilization of counter-stress convex lenses. Because 10 months passed from the most recent accident and the date of the initial optometric examination, it can be assumed that any change in total behavior, reflected in the optometric examination, was the product (or, in this case, the by-product) of utilizing stress-relieving lenses. It is also very conceivable that such lenses—in reducing the tonicity of supporting back musculature—unlocked the persisting hyper-tonicity and imbalance, which caused the vertical deviancy. Thus, the lenses permitted resumption of a more desirable muscular coordination status as well as reduction and elimination of the effect on musculature, which revealed itself as hyperphoria.

What power hath a lens?

Reference
1. Bartley SH. Principles of Perception. 2nd Ed. Harper & Row, 1969:457-458.

CHAPTER 9
Yoked Prisms

Currently, yoked prisms represent the most intriguing, exciting and challenging utilization of lenses within the core of the behavioral aspects of optometry. Frequently clothed in mystery, blue-sky rationalization, and inconsistency, various applications and explanations of the use of yoked prisms have been offered, written about, and discussed in optometric meetings and optometric literature.

Although the very notion of yoked prism utilization had its origins in optometric offices utilizing the behavioral concept, little has been published on the application of yoked prisms from the perspective of a behavioral approach to optometric care. Additionally, most of that which has been presented as well as published (whether from the behavioral concept or otherwise) has focused on the utilization and application of yoked prisms in formalized visual training. The use of yoked prisms in lens prescribing as "Lens Power in Action" has not yet been disclosed. Now is the time.

This author has long incorporated the use of yoked prisms within his practice, both in formalized visual training and in lens prescribing. The use of yoked prisms is both highly selective and very specific; understanding their use is both rational and consistent. Yet, such use can be explained only from a perspective of the *dynamic functional concept of vision.*

The term was coined to differentiate yoked prisms from the more standard utilization of lateral pairs of base-out or base-in prisms and from vertical prism prescribing such as base-up before one eye and base-down before the other. More specifically (and by way of descriptive definition), yoked prisms are pairs of prisms of equal power with bases in the same direction. Thus, we may consider the following four basic sets of yoked prisms: (1) bases-left, (2) bases-right, (3) bases-up, and (4) bases-down. Bases-left yoked prisms are a pair of equal power prisms with the right lens, base-in, and left lens, base-out. Bases-right yoked prisms are the exact opposite. Bases-up yoked prisms are a pair of equal power prisms with both lenses bases-up, and bases-down yoked prisms are the exact opposite.

As stated above, the use of such lenses is highly selective and specific. They are utilized for a specific purpose related to the potential alteration of behavior. Low powers are used. If yoked prisms are utilized, we have the means with our current understanding to determine which base to use. Yet, on the other hand, we have no specific means to determine the degree of power other than professional judgment. All of this will be shared with and explained to the reader as we proceed.

Earlier in this book, it was noted that there are very few facts in the real world, although there are many concepts, theories and notions. Frequently, we are guided by our concepts, theories, and notions. Often, we are guided by a notion in our clinical activity and then we alter this activity, as we no longer subscribe to the notion. On the other hand, we may pursue an activity because it seems to work, although the original notion for the activity is altered and the original rationale is no longer valid.

Consistent with this and related historically to the development and utilization of yoked prisms, this author is reminded of some observations, incorrect simplifications, and inappropriate applications that he made with prisms and yoked prisms more than 25 years ago in formalized visual training. The author at that time noted, when working with vertical dissociating prisms (i.e., base-up before one eye, base-down before the other), that those diplopic images viewed through the base-up were closer and smaller than those viewed through the base-down. This was an exciting revelation at the time. SILO (smaller in, larger out) was experienced and seemed to suggest, based on the assumptions at the time that base-down created a response like that of a plus lens, and vice versa. The observations were very real and consistent; as it turned out, the conclusions were very wrong. We learned the hard way.

During the same period of time, the applied concept of the day associated with visual training was that the first step in visual training was to disorganize the present behavior and then proceed to reorganize. We became aware of the strange and weird physical effects on the body when we created a mismatch with high degrees of yoked lateral prism, such as 15 diopters each lens. And then we asked the patient to move through space, such as walking on a walking board or simply moving about a room. We did such activities for a while using bases-right and then bases-left; the aim was for the patient ultimately to reestablish a match between gravity and what he saw, thus reducing weird body effects, such as body torques.

The rationale was that we were disorganizing the patient. Such use of lenses ceased when we began to appreciate that this particular notion was inappropriate. The concept of disorganization was equivalent to unlearning a pattern of behavior. Admittedly, it was a long while (nearly through the 1950's) before we learned, as W. Gray Walter so aptly stated, "The one thing you cannot learn to do is unlearn; one can only replace patterns of behavior with other patterns of behavior."

It was not until the late 1960's that this author once again began to give serious consideration to (1) the use of yoked prisms in visual training, and (2) prescribing such lenses. The re-involvement, numerous clinical investigations, and applications emerged as a product of continued study, involvement, and a broadening of the dynamic functional concept of vision and all its implications, especially those related to body mechanics.

As an aside, and yet so specifically related, as the author was writing this chapter, the following was brought to his attention: Reuven Kohn-Raz of Hebrew University reported in the British Journal, Early Child Development and Care (1981:7,4) on a study of learning-disabled (LD) children in which he investigated posture. He found a general correlation between poor balance and reading problems. He noted that the same central nervous system mechanics control both the postural functions and the various processes involved in the decoding and interpretation of visual signals and symbols. He noted further that balance was associated with the subcortical areas of the brain and he wondered if investigators were looking in the wrong place for the site of LD problems.

Wouldn't he be excited to know about the behavioral aspects of optometry? Recall that the key difference between the *behavioral concept of vision* and all others has to do with those 20% of retinal fibers leading to lower centers.

In an earlier chapter, Skeffington was quoted as saying that the value of a lens is that it can change orders to the system. It was noted also that a lens does nothing to a person, but a person can do much with a lens. On the other hand, a lens (or pair of lenses) placed before an eye (or pair of eyes) adds to the existing optical mechanism and as a result alters the light distribution or light direction on the retina.

To begin to appreciate the role of yoked prisms, let us first examine what such lenses do to the eye and then, in turn, evaluate what a person does with such a lens combination.

There is absolutely nothing mysterious about the influence of a prism on the light passing through the prism. The light is bent toward the base; and the degree of bend is proportional directly to the power of the prism. The result: that which is viewed is angled (appears displaced) toward the apex of the prism. As an example, when base-right prism is placed before an eye, the light is bent to the right and the object viewed is shifted to the left. The subject must look to the left to continue looking directly at the object with prism in place. In other words, the primary influence of yoked prisms is to effect a movement of the eyes in the direction of the apex of the prism.

Bases-left yoked prisms result in the eyes shifted to the right; bases-up results in the eyes shifted downward; and bases-down result in eyes shifted upward. The critical point being made is that there is a shift in eye position—right, left, up, or down.

The author must request the reader at this time to experiment in order to appreciate the significance and reality of the influence of eye movement on body mechanics and the ultimate value and role of yoked prisms.

Either stand in a well-balanced position or sit on a hard chair. With your eyes gently closed, place your attention on the hip area of your body. Slowly, but forcibly, move your eyes first to the right extreme position and then to the left extreme position. As you continue this, become sensitive to your hip and pelvis positions. Can you feel the hips or pelvis move? What is the movement? Is it in the same direction you move your eyes or in the opposite direction? When you can truly experience the resultant, change to the vertical movement up and down, and again note the rotation of the pelvis. Is it in the same direction as eye movement or opposite?

If you are truly introspective and if you really can be sensitive to yourself, you will discover obviously that the movement in the pelvis and hips is opposite the movement of the eyes. This is basic body mechanics. The real value of yoked prism, in the final analysis, is the influence on orientation. Again, this is an example of what a person can do with a lens. The lens, itself, only can alter the light distribution and/or direction, but the person can alter eye position and body position. Herein lies the significance. It is certainly not mysterious; but it is intriguing and challenging.

Again, refer back to Chapter 6, in which balance mechanics and the resulting center of gravity was discussed. It was noted that the order of commitment of body function related to any physical activity was to come to balance, first, with gravity, and second with the task. From this is derived the center of gravity. The primary center of action lies within the pelvis activity. It was noted also that all ocular defects are reflections of alterations and adaptations in body posture. As the pelvis rotates, the center of gravity shifts. For example, upward rotation of the pelvis shifts the center of gravity forward of the body; a pelvic tilt downward results in the center of gravity moving backward. The pelvis can rotate about the gravitational axis resulting in combinations of lateral and Z-axis shifts as well as vertical changes. The latter is seen in conditions of asymmetry, such as strabismus, amblyopia, and anisometropia.

The specific influence of yoked prisms (and related eye movement) on the pelvis is as follows:

Yoked Prisms	Eye Movement	Pelvis Shift
Bases-up	Down	Tilt upward
Bases-down	Up	Tilt downward
Bases-right	Left	Rotation right
Bases-left	Right	Rotation left

Now, with this information and the influence of yoked prisms on orientation, the reader can appreciate why these lenses must not be utilized indiscriminately and without insight. Such lenses always are used selectively and only when it is determined that alteration of body function is desired and constructive to the program of vision care. In the final analysis, use of such lenses is made when it is deemed both conceivable and desirable to alter body posture. This, in turn, alters the visual process. Although rarely done, such lenses can also be used—not to alter body mechanics—but to permit more effective functioning of an existing asymmetric performance. The latter is considered the compensatory use of yoked prisms as opposed to the more common "therapeutic" utilization. This chapter will consider only the therapeutic utilization in lens prescribing. Use of such lenses in formalized visual training will not be discussed here, but such use may be obvious; appropriate realizations can be derived by the reader from the implications discussed.

The fundamental principle applied in the therapeutic utilization of yoked prisms is similar to that associated with orthodonture or that principle applied to alter bone length. For example, if it is desired to increase the length of a long bone, it is not stretched; on the contrary, it is compressed. In other words, a stress is induced in the direction opposite to that which is ultimately desired. The end result is that the movement or change is in the direction opposite the line of stress. This is a supreme example of the biological principle often quoted by D. B. Harmon, Ph.D., i.e., that an organism grows along a line of stress to reduce stress—the process of adaptation.

When indicated as a potential incorporation in a prescription, yoked prisms are frequently part of a bifocal prescription and worn constantly. Careful monitoring of the patient is required because it is as important to know when to eliminate the yoked prisms from the prescription, as it is to know when to prescribe them. Yoked prisms are prescribed when it is indicated that an alteration of posture is conceivable and constructive to the ultimate change in desired visual behavior. As an example, if the optometric examination evidences movement to myopia, and if yoked prisms benefit is revealed, it will be prescribed in bifocal form along with the appropriate counter-stress plus lens for near.

The specific guidelines for the yoked prisms if indicated as appropriate can be stated as follows:

The yoked prisms that are used are those, which move the person more in the direction of the asymmetry, and, thus, serve to exaggerate the asymmetry. They serve to induce a stress in the direction of the asymmetry and the system will respond to reduce the stress and, thus, alter the asymmetry in the desired direction.

The myopic postural alteration is revealed as a pelvic tilt upward which shifts the center of gravity forward. Bases-up yoked prisms do the same thing. Bases-down would be utilized in cases of adverse hyperopia. Bases-right and bases-left will be prescribed when the asymmetry reveals lateral rotations. For example, any identifiable anisometropia suggests the possible incorporation of lateral yoked prism. The same is true of amblyopia ex anopsia.

Throughout this chapter, the phrase has been used, "when yoked prisms are conceivably valuable, constructive and indicated." The indication and possible constructive value is a derivative or product of the data, clinical observations of the optometric examination, and an evaluation of the information. The asymmetries revealed in the analytical examination, the postural observations made, particularly of head position, and the Polaroid stereo test results with probe yoked-prisms have been most significant to this author.

Earlier in this chapter, the author said that the optometric examination and evaluation will reveal the potential value of yoked prisms, but unfortunately, to this date, we have no specific concrete means to determine appropriate quantitative values as to how much prism. We use low values—generally, no more than 3 or 4 diopters of prism. The general guideline for quantitative value is as follows:

The dioptric value of the yoked prisms should be less than that which the patient is consciously aware of. For example, if bases-up are desired, use one diopter less than that which creates an awareness of space distortion.

It is common to note an improvement on Polaroid stereo tests such as the Wirt and the Randot when the appropriate counter-stress lenses are placed before the eyes.

However, the influence of yoked prisms was revealed to the author some years ago when investigating the performance of a young child who had amblyopia ex anopsia. The child demonstrated complete suppression on all binocular tests, and she had no response on the Wirt test, including the Stereo Fly. Although the author cannot recall what prompted him to investigate, lateral yoked prisms were placed in front of the eyes. With one of the pairs (but not the other), the Stereo Fly jumped out, and she saw the circle protrude in the #3 diamond of the Wirt test. This led the author to conduct additional investigations with many patients; ultimately, insight was derived and conclusions were drawn.

Questions, such as "What in the world do yoked prisms have to do with binocularity?" must arise. Doesn't this lead to a question, such as "What is binocularity?" Hopefully, the reader now will be able to understand the reasons and rationale for "Lens Power in Action" with the background provided in these chapters relative to the visual process and the Behavioral Concept of Vision.

Currently, Polaroid stereo tests provide the best indicators for the use of yoked prisms in lens prescribing, when the total optometric examination suggests the possibility. With the assumption that either the Wirt stereo test or the Randot test has been given the patient and the result noted, the specific guidelines for yoked prisms are as follows:
1. If vertical yoked prisms are suggested, and if:
   a. Bases-up improve performance and/or bases-down reduce performance, prescribe bases-down.
   b. Bases-down improve performance and/or bases-up reduce performance, prescribe bases-up.
2. If lateral yoked prisms are suggested, and if:
   a. Bases-right improve performance and/or bases-left reduce performance, prescribe bases-left.
   b. Bases-left improve performance and/or bases-right reduce performance, prescribe bases-right.

Please note the generality of prescribing yoked prisms. The prisms are used which reduce performance. They induce stress in the direction of the asymmetry. Finally, it should be noted, if yoked prisms are prescribed, they should be removed when they are no longer significant. They are no longer significant when the yoked prisms do not reduce performance or their opposites do not improve performance. Low powered yoked prisms are very potent and they can be used to the patient's benefit, but they must be monitored very closely.

RM, the patient, was 15 years old when he was seen by this author for the first time. He saw clearly with both eyes open, but a recent vision screening at his school revealed poor visual acuity at a distance with the right eye.

Since he was to take driver education, he was concerned about passing the visual requirements for an unrestricted driver's license.

RM had no complaints or symptoms, and he had had no previous vision care. In response to questions about his history, he remarked that reading made him sleepy. However, RM was an excellent student enrolled in a demanding and rigorous high school program. His coordination was reported as excellent, and his major hobby was riding and performing with unicycles.

The eye health investigation revealed no evidence of pathology or abnormality.

The optometric examination data follows:

Unaided visual acuity at far: OD 20/133, OS 20/33, OU 20/29

Unaided visual acuity at near: 20/20 OD, OS and OU; the left eye was of poorer quality

Cover test: Ortho at far and near

Convergence nearpoint: 1 inch, left eye, then right eye deviating out with diplopia reported; recovery at 6 inches

Ocular motility: pursuits were full, without restriction but jerky

Preferred eye: right, but he was left-handed

Head position: tilted left, turned extreme right

Visual abilities: (Telebinocular, DB Series):

    DB10 (pig and dog): both present with suppression
    DB8 (line and ball): suppression
    DB4K (3 balls): 3 balls with suppression
    DB6D (stereopsis): #9
    DB3B (signboards, OD): #3 (29/122 both eyes open; with left eye occluded, #6 (20/60)
    DB2D (signboards, OS): #9 (20/20)
    DB9 (far) (arrow and numbers): #8 steady
    DB9 (near) (arrow and numbers): #1 unstable
    DB5K (3 balls at near): 4 balls in eso

WIRT stereo:
    Without lenses OU: #4
    With bases-left yoked prisms OU: #4
    With bases-right yoked prisms OU: #2
    With -1.25 OD and Plano OS: #4

Before listing the analytical sequence data, the following comments on the phoria findings are necessary. The author has long thought it necessary to routinely do both a right eye and left eye phoria on #15B (phoria through the fused cross cylinder). A right eye phoria is the phoria measurement with the patient directed to fixate the right eye's target and reporting when there is alignment; a left eye phoria is the opposite. Also routinely, all phoria measurements are performed, both right eye fixing and left eye fixing, when anisometropia or antimetropia exists. This is reflected in the following collection of data. Unless specific instructions are given for patient fixation, the target associated with the preferred eye will be that fixated during these measurements.

The Analytical Sequence:

#3 (habitual distance phoria)	OD 5 eso OS 6 eso
#13A (habitual near phoria)	OD 6 eso OS 6 eso
#4 (retinoscopy)	OD -0.75 sphere OS Plano
#5 (retinoscopy at 20 inches)	OD +0.75 sphere OS +2.25 sphere
#7 (subjective)	OD -1.25 sphere OS +0.25 -0.25 x 180
#8 (phoria through #7)	OD 6 eso OS 5 eso

Control	#7	Plano OU
#9 (base out blur)	X	X
#10 (base out break/recovery)	24/15	25/14
#11 (base in break/recovery)	6/2	7/3

#12 (vertical phoria)--1 right hyper

#13B (near phoria through #7)--Not done

#14A (unfused cross cylinder)	OD Plano OS +1.75 w/cyl.
#15A (phoria through #14A)	OD 2 exo OS 5 exo

#14B (fused cross cylinder)   OD Plano
                              OS +1.75 w/cyl.

#15B (phoria through #14B)   OD 2 exo
                              OS 4 exo

    (Control at near: Plano)

#16A (base out blur)--X   #16B (base our break/recovery)--24/14

#17A (base in blur)--X   #17B (base in break/recovery)--19/10

#18 (vertical phoria)--Ortho

#19 (amplitude of accommodation) 4.25

#20 (minus lens to blur out)-- -3.00

#21 (plus lens to blur out)--+3.00

Stresspoint retinoscopy: OU +1.00 spheres provided best balance

An evaluation of the collected data and information revealed the embedded syndrome of the stress-induced visual dysfunction, the major adaptation being environmentally influenced anisometropic myopia. This resulted in asymmetric functioning.

"He Had Everything to Gain and Nothing to Lose."

The patient and his parents were informed of the possible alternatives of optometric care that could be provided. The conventional approach simply would have been to provide compensatory lenses equivalent to the #7 (subjective) or, possibly, to do nothing immediately and wait until he was more myopic, with an obvious restriction in distance visual acuity and then provide compensatory lenses. The alternative was the behavioral approach —the therapeutic use of lenses.

Such lenses would be in dual focus form and would be used initially as constantly as possible or, at a minimum, during all waking hours spent indoors. He would be programmed for a reevaluation examination in three months. Formal visual training was discussed as an additional alternative but, in view of his status and needs, only in order to achieve benefits beyond what could be derived from the therapeutic use of lenses.

The behavioral approach was selected by the patient and his parents, and the prescription provided was: OU Plano, 4 bases-right yoked prisms, add +1.00 D-35 bifocals, the segment height at level of lower edge of pupils.

The behavioral alternative was requested because the potential benefits to be gained from the use of these therapeutic lenses more appropriately represented the needs and desires of the patient. Obviously, he was aware of the difference in visual acuity of the two eyes; likewise, he was not aware of any restriction with both eyes open. Additionally, he was not interested in the possibility of becoming more myopic overall. Thus, when it was suggested (and predicted) that possible reduction of the asymmetry, possible reduction and/or alleviation of the myopia, and control against additional adverse maladaptation could be anticipated as products of utilizing therapeutic lenses, the behavioral approach unquestionably was the choice. He had everything to gain and nothing to lose.

RM was unable to return for his progress case study until October because of scheduling problems. He reported then that he used his glasses as constantly as possible and, once again, he was unaware of any problems.

The significant findings revealed were as follows:

Unaided visual acuity at far: OD 20/89, OS 20/25, OU 20/22

Unaided visual acuity at near: OD, OS and OU 20/20

Convergence nearpoint: 1 inch, right eye deviating with diplopia reported: recovery at 4 inches

Ocular motility: pursuit movements full and jerky

Telebinocular:

DB6D (stereopsis): #9
DB3D (signboards, OD): #8 (20/33) no improvement with occlusion of left eye

The Analytical findings:

#3 (habitual distance phoria)	OD 8 eso OS 4 eso
#13A (habitual near phoria)	OD 7 eso OS 12 eso
#4 (retinoscopy)	OD -1.00 sphere OS +0.25 -0.50 x 180
#5 (retinoscopy at 20 inches)	OD +1.25 sphere OS +2.50 -0.50 x 180
#7 (subjective)	OD -0.75 sphere OS +0.25
#8 (phoria through #7)	OD 5 eso OS 3 eso

(Control at far: OU Plano)

#9 (base out blur)--X

#10 (base out break/recovery)--24/14

#11 (base in break/recovery)--10/3

#12 (vertical phoria)--Ortho
 (Control at near: OU +1.00 sphere)

#13B (near phoria through #7)   OD 1 eso
                                                     OS 4 eso

#16AB (base out blur/break/recovery)--X/25/10

#17AB (base in blur/break/recovery)--X/26/17

Stresspoint retinoscopy: OU +1.00 spheres provided best balance

WIRT stereo:
 With Plano OU: #5
 With +1.00 sphere OU: #5
 With +1.00 sphere and bases-left yoked prisms OU: #5
 With +1.00 sphere and bases-right yoked prisms OU: #4

Changes in function were noted and reported to the patient, and he was informed that the data suggested he still was in the process of changing. Therefore, it was recommended that appropriate use of the lenses be continued. He was programmed to return for his next progress case study in four months.

The next office visit was delayed until March, due to scheduling difficulties. He reported that he had continued to use the lenses as instructed. Again, he reported no problems or symptoms. The big news, however, was that he passed his driver's test vision requirements and he was now driving. The salient findings were as follows:

Unaided visual acuity at far: OD 20/53, OS 20/20, OU 20/20

Convergence nearpoint: to the nose (no break)

Ocular motility: pursuit movements were smooth

The Analytical findings:

#3 (habitual distance phoria)   OD 3 eso
                                                     OS 3 eso

#13A (habitual near phoria)   OD 5 eso
                                                     OS 6 eso

#4 (retinoscopy)   OD -0.50 -0.50 x 90
                                               OS Plano

#5 (retinoscopy at 20 inches)   OD +1.50 -0.50 x 90
                                               OS +2.00 sphere

#7 (subjective)   OD -0.75
                                               OS +0.25

    (Control at far: OU Plano)

#9 (base out blur)--X

#10 (base out break/recovery)--26/23

#11 (base in break/recovery)--9/6
    (Control at near: OU +1.00 sphere)

#13B (near phoria through #7)   OD 1 exo
                                               OS 2 eso

#16AB (base out blur/break/recovery)--X/22/14

#17AB (base in blur/break/recovery)--28/23

Stresspoint retinoscopy: OU +1.00 spheres provided best balance

WIRT stereo:
    With Plano OU: #9
    With +1.00 sphere OU: #9
    With +1.00 sphere and bases-left yoked prisms OU: #9
    With +1.00 sphere and bases-right yoked prisms OU: #7

RM attained his goal ... an unrestricted driver's license, and he avoided additional myopic progression.

The data revealed more changes in visual behavior and performance as a product of the additional time utilizing the therapeutic lenses. RM attained his goal, which was to have an unrestricted driver's license, and he avoided additional myopic progression. The myopia was reduced; distance visual acuity improved, and the data suggested he had stabilized. This had been predicted when the behavioral alternative was presented. The final product resulted from the patient's cooperation in utilizing the lenses properly.

Although someone might argue that the patient is deprived by not having a minus lens to compensate for the right eye's remaining myopia, the evidence suggests no such deprivation. He is binocular; he is deriving the benefits afforded by the binocular inputs. From the behavioral point of view, there is no constructive value to RM in the use of a minus lens for general functioning.

In view of this apparent stabilization, RM was instructed, following the progress case study, to continue the use of the lenses for all near-centered activities, primarily as a controlling and protecting means now, rather than as a therapeutic one, which originally was the case. The prescription was not altered to eliminate the bases-right yoked prisms because the data indicated that it was constructive and significant. The WIRT stereo test demonstrated that the bases-right yoked prisms still reduced the response, which, is one of the prime indicators for use of yoked prisms.

The programming for RM's vision care continued. He was seen again for reevaluation examinations two times the following year. On each of these occasions, the results were similar to the former progress case study. No changes were made either in the prescription or in the recommended use of the lenses.

RM's next programmed office visit was scheduled for after he had completed the first semester of his freshman year of college. If his performance remains as before, he will then be programmed for an annual complete examination. The yoked prisms will be removed from the prescription only if they are no longer significant. For example, they will be eliminated immediately when they no longer deprecate the WIRT stereo test. The plus lens element of the prescription relieves the stress of near-centered demands and it is essential for control and protection. It will be altered only if the stresspoint retinoscopy procedure indicates it should be.

Experience demonstrates that it is absolutely essential to monitor patient behavior and performance closely, and perhaps even more than usual when using yoked prisms. There are times when yoked prisms should be used to alter performance in the desired direction. However, there are times when they should not be used. Yoked prisms are a powerful tool, which can directly affect posturing mechanisms and alter orientation. The general rule is that they are used when the potential change to achieving desired performance outweighs the possible negative influences on posture. It is important to guard against undesired responses or changes.

Monitoring is a must

This section reports optometric care of a child using lenses and yoked prisms over a more than two-year period. Emphasis is placed on the need to periodically assess, monitor and control patients' performance when using yoked prisms, as well as to observe and try to modify patients' posture, when appropriate.

MF, a 9-year-old girl, was seen for an examination on May 31. She had no complaints or symptoms of discomfort. MF was an excellent student and she reported no difficulty seeing clearly. The eye health screening was negative. The significant optometric findings were as follows:

Unaided visual acuity at far: OD 20/20, OS 20/160, OU 20/20

Unaided visual acuity at near: OD, OS, OU 20/20

Ocular motility: pursuits were smooth and fixations accurate

Convergence nearpoint: to nose

Asymmetry noted: head turned left, eyes turned right

The Analytical Sequence:

#3 (habitual distance phoria)	OD 1 exo OS 1 exo
#13A (habitual near phoria)	OD 3 exo OS 8 exo
#4 (retinoscopy)	OD Plano OS -1.25 sphere
#5 (retinoscopy at 20 inches)	OD +1.50 sphere OS +0.50 sphere
#7 (subjective)	OD Plano OS -1.25 sphere
#8 (phoria through #7)	OD 1 exo OS Ortho

(Control at far: OU Plano)

#9 (base out blur)--X

#10 (base out break/recovery)--16/2

#11 (base in break/recovery)--7/3

#14A (unfused cross cylinder)	OD +1.50 OS +0.50
#15A (phoria through #14A)	OD 15 exo OS 9 exo

(Control at near: OU +0.75 sphere)

#16A (base out blur)--X   #16B (base out break/recovery)--11/-2

#17A (base in blur)--X   #17B (base in break/recovery)--20/13

WIRT Stereo:
- With Plano OU: #8
- With +0.75 sphere OU: #9
- With Plano, bases-right yoked prisms OU: #8
- With Plano, bases-left yoked prisms OU: #6

Stresspoint retinoscopy: OU +0.75 sphere provides best balance

Although there were no symptoms, complaints or adverse observations by the child or her parents, the parents were interested in a behavioral approach to optometric care. (The child was most cooperative.) The difference in the distance visual acuity of the two eyes was obvious both to the parents and the young girl.

They were told that MF demonstrated a stress-induced visual problem in which myopia emerged in the left eye. Also, she probably was in the process of moving into more myopia of both eyes as a total response. The asymmetry revealed in the visual system was reflected in the asymmetry of the body.

Goals, desires and needs were discussed and established. It was unnecessary (and undesirable) to provide any form of compensatory lenses because there was no impairment or limitation in general visual acuity. On the other hand, it was desirable to prevent additional myopia from emerging, and to alter and, hopefully, to reduce the asymmetry. It was agreed that the prescribed program of vision care was temporary constant-wear lenses. The prescription given her was: OU Plano, 4 bases-left yoked prisms, add +0.75, using executive bifocals. A progress case study was planned for October. This would enable her to use the lenses throughout the summer when school pressures were reduced. She would be seen again after she was a few weeks into the next school semester.

She returned for her reevaluation examination, as scheduled, in October. Her parents reported that she was most cooperative and that she used the glasses as prescribed. Again, there was no report of any symptoms or complaints. The optometric data revealed significant benefits and rewards as a product of behavioral optometric care. The significant findings were as follows:

Unaided visual acuity at far: OD 20/20, OS 20/62, OU 20/20

#3 (habitual distance phoria)   OD 1 eso
                                                  OS 1 exo

#13A (habitual near phoria) (Plano) OD 2 eso
                                                        OS 2 eso

#4 (retinoscopy)   OD Plano
                                           OS -0.75 sphere

#5 (retinoscopy at 20 inches)   OD +1.75 sphere
                                           OS +0.75 sphere

#7 (subjective)   OD +0.25 sphere
                                           OS -0.75 sphere

#8 (phoria through #7)   OD 1 eso
                                           OS Ortho

Control	Plano	#7 (subjective)
#10 (base out break/recovery)	16/2	17/4
#11 (base in break/recovery)	6/2	7/2

(Control at near: OU +0.75 sphere)

#13B (near phoria through #7)   OD 1 exo
                                              OS 6 eso

#16B (base out break/recovery)--23/9

#17B (base in break/recovery)--19/12

WIRT Stereo:
    With Plano OU: #9
    With +0.75 sphere OU: #9
    With Plano, bases-right yoked prisms OU: #9
    With Plano, bases-left yoked prisms OU: #3

Stresspoint retinoscopy: OU +0.75 sphere provides best balance

Appraisal of the data revealed significant improvement in the distance visual acuity and reduced myopia (.50 diopter) in the left eye as well as a shift to plus in the right eye at distance. There was a reduction of the asymmetry and a dramatic change in the #16B (base out break/recovery at near). Stresspoint retinoscopy continued to demonstrate the importance of the equal plus at near. The WIRT stereo suggested definitively that the same therapeutic program of constant lens use be continued because she appeared to be still in process of improvement. She was programmed to return in three months for her next progress case study.

MF and her family moved from the area before there was an opportunity to see her for the next programmed office visit. She was referred to a colleague who could continue the behavioral approach to her optometric care. She was reexamined by the colleague the following spring and it was reported that the distance visual acuity of the left eye improved with additional reduction in the myopia. There was less asymmetry, and there no longer was a difference between bases-right and bases-left yoked prism findings on the WIRT stereo test. The visual performance was stable. The yoked prisms were removed from her prescription, and she was given OU Plano, Add +0.75 to be worn for all near-centered activity for purposes of protection and control.

Latest reports have confirmed the continued stability of her visual performance and function.

The importance of careful and controlled monitoring of patient performance, especially when utilizing yoked prisms, has already been emphasized. Indeed, MF's case was very rewarding; but her condition prior to her examination when she was 9 years old accentuated the importance of patient control and monitoring.

Actually, MF was seen initially by the author for her first complete optometric examination when she was 7 years old, and she was in second grade. Although she was not having major academic problems, the school reported that she had difficulty following directions. Also, she complained of severe periodic parietal headaches. The parents noted no evidence of sight problems. The investigation of eye health was negative. There was no restriction, limitation or distortion of pursuit and fixation eye movement. Convergence nearpoint was to the nose. The optometric findings were as follows:

Unaided visual acuity at far: OD 20/25, OS 20/20, OU poor 20/20

Unaided visual acuity at near: OD, OS, OU 20/20

Visual Abilities (Telebinocular, DB series):
    DB10 (pig and dog): both present
    DB4K (3 balls): 3 balls with suppression
    DB6D (stereopsis): #12
    DB3 (signboards OD): 20/45 (20/33 with left eye occluded)
    DB2 (signboards OS): 20/18
    DB9 (far—arrow and numbers): #8
    DB9 (near—arrow and numbers): #4
    DB5K (3 balls at near): 3 balls with suppression

WIRT Stereo:
    OU Plano: #9
    OU Plano with bases-up yoked prisms: #8

The Analytical Sequence:

#3 (habitual distance phoria)--Ortho   #13A (habitual near phoria) Ortho

#4 (retinoscopy)	OD Plano
	OS -0.50 sphere
#5 (retinoscopy at 20 inches)	OD +1.75
	OS +1.25
#7 (subjective)	OD +0.50 sphere 20/20
	OS +0.25 sphere 20/25

#8 (phoria through #7)--1 exo

#10 (base out break/recovery)--17/0

#11 (base in break/recovery)--8/2

#13B (near phoria through #7)--2 exo

#14A & B (unfused and fused cross cylinder)--No significant responses (Control at near: OU Plano)

#16B (base out break/recovery)--17/2

#17B (base in break/recovery)--21/4

#20 (minus lens to blur out)-- -1.50

#21 (plus lens to blur out)--+2.25

Stresspoint retinoscopy: OU +0.75 sphere provided best balance

Analysis of the data revealed the non-embedded syndrome of stress-induced visual dysfunction, which probably created initial disturbance in information processing as well as the headache discomforts. It was suspected that she was in the process of moving into myopia. It was recommended that she be given counter-stress therapeutic lenses in dual focus form to be used indoors always. This ensured that such lenses would be used for all close work. The prescription was OU Plano, 4 bases-up yoked prisms, Add +0.75, executive bifocals. She was programmed to return in two months for a reevaluation examination.

However, numerous problems arose which prevented her from being seen for the scheduled progress case study. Instead, she was scheduled and seen nine months later. It was reported that she used the glasses as prescribed. She reported no problems in learning and she did not have any headaches. In fact, she never complained of headaches once she began use of the lenses.

The significant data follow:

Unaided visual acuity at far: OD poor 20/20, OS slow 20/25, OU 20/20

The Analytical Sequence:

#13A (habitual near phoria through Plano)--½ exo

#4 (retinoscopy)	OD +0.25 sphere OS -0.25 sphere
#5 (retinoscopy at 20 inches)	OD +1.75 sphere OS +1.25 sphere
#7 (subjective)	OD +0.25 sphere 20/20 OS Plano poor 20/20

    (Note: -0.50, good 20/20)

#8 (phoria through #7)--Ortho

#10 (base out break/recovery)--17/4

#11 (base in break/recovery)-8/3

#13B (near phoria through OU +0.75 sphere)--2 exo
    (Control at near: OU +0.75 sphere)

#16B (base out break/recovery)--19/4

#17B (base in break/recovery)--21/4

#20 (minus lens to blur out)-- -3.50

WIRT Stereo:
    With Plano OU: #9
    With +0.75 OU: #9
    With +0.75, 4 bases-up yoked prisms OU: #8

Stresspoint retinoscopy: OU +0.75 provided best balance

The parents were pleased and the patient was both comfortable and cooperative. However, the examiner was still concerned. The myopia tendency and drive persisted; in fact, it was even more evidenced. But, there was no suggestion at the time to change the prescription. She was instructed to continue to use the lenses as much of the time as possible. The next office visit was scheduled for the following February.

MF was reexamined in February, as preprogrammed. Once again, she proved to be cooperative. She had used the glasses as recommended. She had no discomfort or complaints, and she saw clearly. However, the data were alarming in that significant evidence of asymmetric performance was revealed for the first time. The findings were as follows:

Unaided visual acuity at far: OD 20/20, OS 20/50, OU 20/20

Unaided visual acuity at near: OD, OS, OU 20/20

Asymmetry revealed: when looking straight ahead, head was turned left and eyes turned right

The Analytical Sequence:

#3 (habitual distance phoria)   OD Ortho
                                OS 1 exo

#13A (habitual near phoria through Plano) OD 1 eso
                                OS 1 ½ exo

#4 (retinoscopy)   OD Plano
                                OS -0.75 sphere

#5 (retinoscopy at 20 inches)   OD +1.75 sphere
                                OS +1.00 sphere

#7 (subjective)   OD +0.25 sphere 20/20
                                OS -0.75 sphere 20/20

#8 (phoria through #7)   OD Ortho
                                OS Ortho

   (Control at far: OU Plano)

#10 (base out break/recovery)--13/2

#11 (base in break/recovery)--7/2

#13B (near phoria through OU +0.75)
                                OD Ortho
                                OS 5 exo

#14A (unfused cross cylinder)   OD +2.25
                                OS +1.50

#15A (phoria through #14A)   OD 15 exo
                                OS 15 exo
   (Control at near)   OU +0.75 sphere)

#16B (base out break/recovery)--16/2

#17B (base in break/recovery)--21/10

#20 (positive relative accommodation)-- -3.00

WIRT Stereo:
  With Plano OU: #9
  With +0.75: #9
  With +0.75, bases-up yoked prisms OU: #6
  With +0.75, bases-down yoked prisms OU: #9
  With +0.75, bases-right yoked prisms OU: #9
  With +0.75, bases-left yoked prisms OU: #6

Stresspoint retinoscopy: OU +0.75 sphere provided best balance

MF was given the Harmon Square test because the asymmetry was revealed so obviously.

In brief review, the test is as follows: The patient is seated at the appropriate height desk and chair and given a piece of paper and a pencil. The patient is asked to make a row of squares across the paper, as good squares as possible, one after another, as many as possible, in the patient's normal size handwriting, as rapidly as can be done. Under these circumstances, the patient will assume a habitual postural approach to a handwriting task.

The posture and the quality of the squares are observed. If the habitual posture is other than the best-balanced posture and/or if the squares are distorted, the test is repeated with the patient placed in the best-balanced posture for a writing task.

The difference in the quality of the squares is noted. If the squares are more symmetrical in the best-balanced posture than in the habitual posture, a non-embedded asymmetric performance is indicated and appropriate recommendations for changes in the postural approach to a handwriting task are in order. If the converse is true, or if the squares are similar to the habitual position, the behavior is more embedded and it may not be wise to alter the postural approach.

For specific reference to balanced and desirable postural approaches to writing activities, the reader is referred to publications available from the Optometric Extension Program Foundation, one for study, "Vision, Body Mechanics, and Performance," by Darell Boyd Harmon, Ph.D., and two for study and handing to parents or patients, (1) "Visual Hygiene—Effective Visual Hygiene Makes Learning and Earning Easier," and (2) "Easier and More Productive Study and Desk Work," by A. W. Francke, O.D., and W. J. Kaplan, O.D.

MF was right-handed. The initial test of Harmon Squares in her habitual posture revealed squares, which, in reality, were rectangular—the long axis in the horizontal meridian. With her posture altered to that compatible for a right-handed person (that is, placed in best balance with body turned to the left of the desk so that her left elbow was off the desk top) the squares clearly were symmetrically square.

From this evidence (and with great hopes and expectations), she was instructed to continue the use of the therapeutic lenses, as before, and to consistently as possible control her handwriting postural approach on the desk or table top both in school and at home. The proper postural approach was demonstrated to and experienced by MF and her parents. Additionally, based on the total data at hand, it was suggested to the parents that MF's prescription probably would be modified at the time of the next programmed office visit if the postural approach alone did not alleviate the asymmetric performance. She was scheduled to return for the next progress case study three months later. This was the May examination cited earlier in this chapter.

A further review of the data from that May reevaluation examination revealed continued movement into greater and more manifest asymmetric performance, with increased myopia of the left eye and a further reduction of visual acuity despite the postural control which was added to her program of care. Ultimately, stabilization and improvement in performance emerged when lateral yoked prisms were incorporated into the therapeutic prescription along with the postural controls.

However, this author (and examiner) was concerned with questions such as:

1. Why didn't the examiner see evidence of a need for lateral prisms earlier?
2. Did the patient use the initial prescription with the bases-up yoked prisms too long?
3. If the patient had been seen as initially desired following the original examination when she was 7 years old, instead of being delayed until October of the following year, would there have been reason to have removed the bases-up yoked prisms?

All of these questions relate to the absolute need to control and to monitor performance as carefully as possible when attempting to alter performance with lenses. This applies to ALL patients and parents (in the case of children) in order to obtain maximum benefits and to avoid lingering questions and concerns like those suggested above. To provide the best in behavioral optometric care, a controlled program of vision care is an absolute must.

The almost myope

The fundamental purpose for the use of yoked prisms is to alter orientation by alteration of the body's posturing mechanisms. Recall that the posture of the myope causes the center of gravity to be shifted forward; this is reflected as a pelvic tilt upward. The therapeutic directive is to use the yoked prism, which drives the system in the direction of its deviancy.

In the case of myopia, this directive is satisfied by the application of bases-up yoked prisms, which, in the final analysis, induce an exaggeration of a pelvic tilt upward and a shift of the center of gravity further forward. If free to do so, the system will respond to this induced stress in the opposite direction. This will reduce the stress, reduce the pelvic tilt and shift the center of gravity backward.

LD was seen by this author for her first optometric examination when she was 16 years old and in the 10th grade. She had always been a good student with no learning problems. She read quite a bit and she was unaware of any problems in her reading efficiency. Her movement coordination was reported excellent; she was very involved in sports, such as tennis and soccer. However, she was aware since the beginning of the current school semester of some difficulty seeing the chalkboards in class. She reported that the chalkboards blurred and that she squinted in order to see them. Additionally, she was aware of a delay in "focus" when she shifted from near to far.

The investigation of eye health revealed no evidence of pathology or abnormality.

The optometric examination data were as follows:

Unaided visual acuity at far and near: OD, OS and OU 20/20

Cover test: Ortho at far and near

Convergence nearpoint: 2 inches, left eye deviating out with diplopia reported; recovery at 6 inches

Ocular motility: pursuits were full without restriction, but jerky and spastic; fixation near to far was poor

Preferred eye and hand: right

Visual Abilities (Telebinocular DB series):
    DB10 (pig and dog): both present with suppression
    DB8   (line and ball): suppression
    DB4K (3 balls): 3 balls with suppression
    DB6D (stereopsis): #12

BU 21: (stereo/suppression test) patient suppressed

DB3D (signboards, right eye): #8 (20/20) both eyes open; #10 with left eye occluded

DB2D (signboards, left eye): #9 (20/17)

DB9 (far) (arrow and numbers) #10 steady

DB9 (near) (arrow and numbers) #2
                ½ unsteady

DB5K (3 balls at near): 3 balls, unstable and suppression

Titmus Polaroid Stereo test: with Plano #9, with bases-up yoked prisms, #7

The Analytical Sequence:

#3 (habitual distance phoria)--1 exo   #13A (habitual near phoria)--1 eso

#4 (retinoscopy)	OD -0.25 -0.50 X 90
	OS -0.25 -0.25 X 90
#5 (retinoscopy at 20 inches)	OD +1.50 -0.50 X 90
	OS +1.75 -0.25 X 90
#7 (subjective)	OD +0.25 -0.50 X 100
	OS Plano

#8 (phoria through #7)--1 exo
   (Control at far: OU Plano)

#9 (base out blur)--16

#10 (base out break/recovery)--18/9

#11 (base in break/recovery)--6/3

#12 (vertical phoria)--Ortho

#13B (near phoria through #7)--Ortho

#14A (unfused cross cylinder)   OD +0.75 with cylinder
                                          OS +0.50 sphere

#15A (phoria through #14A)--2 exo

#14B (fused cross cylinder)   OD +0.50 with cylinder
                                        OS +0.25 sphere

#15B (phoria through #14B)--2 exo right and left
   (Control at near: OU Plano)

#16A (base out blur)--X   #16B (base out break/recovery)--13/4

#17A (base in blur)--X   #17B (base in break/recovery)--14/11

#19 (amplitude of accommodation)--6.25

#20 (minus lens to blur out)-- -3.25

#21 (plus lens to blur out)--+3.00

Stresspoint Retinoscopy: OU +0.75 spheres provided best balance

An evaluation of the collected data and information revealed the partially non-embedded syndrome of the stress-induced visual dysfunction with apparent movement of adaptation into myopia. Although the examination revealed no impairment in visual acuity, the data confirmed her periodic difficulty seeing the chalkboards. It seemed very likely at this stage of response to stress and adaptation that she manifested myopia when under demand at school. This examination occurred during her winter vacation from school.

LD and her parents were informed of her visual status and the alternatives of optometric care.

The conventional approach would have been to do nothing and wait for a greater and more significant manifestation of the myopia; at that time she could be provided with compensatory lenses. At the other extreme, formalized visual training could be provided. However, this examiner found no revealed needs or reasons for visual training at this time.

(The reader should be reminded that this author firmly holds to the notion that every human being can profit from formalized visual training. But not everyone is in need of the benefits to be derived as a product of developing a more effective and efficient visual system. This author further holds to the principle that the patient—in order to be accepted for visual training—must have clearly identified vision-related needs that cannot be satisfied through a more simple and positive optometric approach to vision care.)

Analysis of the data and her needs revealed that Laura did not fit the category of acceptability for visual training at the time. The chances were great that her needs could be satisfied through the more simple yet positive approach of LENS POWER.

The recommended alternative, which Laura accepted, was the use of bifocal lenses to be worn as constantly as possible, the minimal use being all indoors (school, home, etc.) while awake. The prescription was: OU Plano with 4 bases-up yoked prisms, add +0.75, executive bifocals. She was also programmed to return for a reevaluation examination in two months.

She did not get her glasses until mid-January, and she was scheduled for the progress case study in March. However, complications such as weather, health, and scheduling prevented her from being seen again until the afternoon of April 23rd after a full day of school.

The following are the results of that office visit:

LD used the glasses as prescribed. She tended to wear them constantly, with the exception of sports activities. She did not experience any discomfort; most importantly, she forgot that she initially had problems seeing chalkboards. The optometric findings were as follows:

Unaided visual acuity at far: OD 20/22, OS 20/20, OU 20/20

Unaided visual acuity at near: OD, OS and OU 20/20

Convergence nearpoint: 2 inches, left eye deviating out with diplopia; recovery at 6 inches

Ocular motility: pursuit movements were full and slightly jerky; fixations were accurate

Analytical findings:
#3 (habitual distance phoria)--2 eso   #13A (habitual near phoria)--2 eso (Plano)

#4 (retinoscopy)   OU +0.25 -0.50 X 90

#5 (retinoscopy at 20 inches)   OU +1.75 -0.50 X 90

#7 (subjective)--OU Plano

#8 (phoria through #7)--2 eso

#9 (base out blur)--16

#10 (base out break/recovery)--19/9

#11 (base in break/recovery)--8/4
   (Control at near: OU +0.75)

#13B (near phoria through control)--4 exo

#16A (base out blur)--X   #16B (base out break/recovery)--17/6

#17B (base in break/recovery)--16/12

Titmus Polaroid stereo test
   With Plano OU: #9
   With OU +0.75 OU: #9
   With bases-up yoked prisms OU: #8

Stresspoint Retinoscopy: OU +0.75 sphere provided best balance

The following observations related to the data were significant:

1. Although LD reported no awareness of blur, the visual acuity of the right eye was less than 20/20; remember, this office visit took place after a full day of school.
2. The #7 was now OU Plano; neither minus sphere nor cylinder was revealed. In fact, behind the phoropter, with Plano, she had 20/20 with right eye.
3. Bases-up yoked prisms still reduced the performance on the Polaroid stereo test, but not as much as originally.

There was nothing to indicate the necessity for any change in the prescription. LD was instructed to continue as before the use of her glasses throughout the remainder of the semester. It was recommended that she use the lenses minimally for near-centered activity, and, preferably, constantly when indoors during the forthcoming summer vacation period.

LD returned for her scheduled reevaluation examination in September. Now in the 11th grade, the school year was only three weeks old. She had continued to use the glasses as recommended and reported no awareness of any problems. This appointment also was scheduled for the afternoon after a day of school. The data were as follows:

Unaided visual acuity at far and near: OD, OS and OU 20/20

Convergence nearpoint: 2 inches, left eye deviating out with diplopia reported; recovery at 5 inches

Ocular motility: pursuit movements were full and smooth

Analytical findings:
#3 (habitual distance phoria)--1 exo   #13A (habitual near phoria)--2 exo (Plano)

#4 (retinoscopy)--OU +0.25 sphere

#5 (retinoscopy at 20 inches)--OU +2.00 sphere

#7 (subjective)--OU +0.50 sphere

#8 (phoria through #7)--1 exo
   (Control at far: OU Plano)

#9 (base out blur)--X

#10 (base out break/recovery)--17/7

#11 (base in break/recovery)--9/5

#13B 4 exo (near phoria through OU +0.75 sphere)

#14A (unfused cross cylinder)--OU +0.50

#15A (phoria through #14A)--8 exo

#14B (fused cross cylinder)--OU +0.50

#15B (phoria through #14B)--4 exo
(Control at near: OU +0.75 sphere)

#16B (base out break/recovery)--16/8

#17A (base in blur)-X   #17B (base in break/recovery)--17/13

Titmus Polaroid stereo test: with Plano, #9; with OU +0.75 sphere, #9; with bases-up yoked prisms, #9

Stresspoint Retinoscopy: OU +0.75 sphere provided best balance

The data of this progress case study revealed significant physiological changes. Most importantly, the #7 (subjective) was now in plus, normal hyperopia and there was no decrement in response on the Polaroid stereo test with bases-up yoked prisms.

Recall the definition of a visual problem—an unsatisfied vision-related personal need. This new data revealed that LD had no visual problem; further, the data revealed no significant inadequacy or disability. Because the initial goals were reached and satisfied, the initial purpose and program of optometric care could be concluded.

Thus, the following was recommended:

1. The prescription was changed to OU Plano, add +0.75. The yoked prisms were dropped from the prescription.
2. The glasses were to be used for all visually near-centered activity and they should be used constantly in school and at home, if desired, so as to assure appropriate near-centered use.
3. She was programmed to return in six months for the next progress case study. If all is satisfactory at that time, Laura will be programmed for an annual complete optometric examination. This programming will continue unless additional needs are identified.

The analytical data of the three visits are listed below for your convenience to compare the data from one office visit to the next.

	12/29	4/23	9/16
#3 (habitual phoria distance)	1 exo	2 eso	1 exo
#13A (habitual phoria near)	1 eso	2 eso (plano)	2 exo (plano)
#4 (retinoscopy)	OD -0.25 -0.50 X 90 OS -0.25 -0.25 X 90	OD +0.25 -0.50 X 90 OS +0.25 -0.50 X 90	OD +0.25 sphere OS +0.25 sphere
#5 (retinoscopy at 20 inches)	OD +1.50 -0.50 X 90 OS +1.75 -0.25 X 90	OD +1.75 -0.50 X 90 OS +1.75 -0.50 X 90	OD +2.00 sphere OS +2.00 sphere
#7 (subjective)	OD +0.25 -0.50 X 100 OS Plano	OD Plano OS Plano	OD +0.50 sphere OS +0.50 sphere
#8 (phoria through #7)	1 exo	2 eso	1 exo
Control at far	OU Plano	OU Plano	OU Plano
#9 (base out blur)	16	16	X
#10 (base out break/recovery)	18/9	19/9	17/7
#11 (base in break/recovery)	6/3	8/4	9/5
#12 (vertical phoria)	Ortho	Ortho	Ortho
#13B (near phoria through #7)	Ortho	4 exo (OU +0.75)	4 exo (OU +0.75)
#14A (unfused cross cylinder)	OD +0.75 with cylinder OS +0.50 sphere	OD +0.50 sphere OS +0.50 sphere	
#15A (phoria through #14A)	2 exo	8 exo	
#14B (fused cross cylinder)	OD +0.50 with cylinder OS +0.25 sphere	OD +0.50 sphere OS +0.50 sphere	
#15B (phoria through #14B)	2 exo	2 exo	
Control at near	OU Plano	OU +0.75 sphere	OU +0.75 sphere
#16A (base out blur)	X	X	X
#16B (base out break/recover)	13/4	17/6	16/8
#17A (base in blur)	X	X	X

#17B (base in break/recovery)	14/11	16/12	17/13
#19 (amplitude of accommodation)	6.25		
#20 (positive relative accommodation)	-3.25		
#21 (negative relative accommodation)	+3.00		
Stresspoint Retinoscopy	#9	#9	#9
Titmus Polaroid with +0.75	#9	#9	
Titmus Polaroid Base-up Yoked	#7	#8	#9

Further considerations of yoked prisms

This author collaborated with Darell Boyd Harmon, Ph.D., on a study related to visual function and body mechanics. Entitled "A Preliminary Report on a Study of Eye Preference, Certain Body Mechanics and Visual Problems," the study was published in Learning Disorders, Volume 2 (Jerome Hellmuth, Editor, Special Child Publications, Seattle, WA.).

Data for the study were collected from 100 consecutive patients seen in the author's office. The data confirmed and broadened Dr. Harmon's appreciation of vision and body mechanics. For a complete background on this study, the reader is referred to the source cited above.

One factor considered in the study was the relationship of patients' head turn to their refractive status and asymmetry in posture. Specifically, a patient's attention was fixated on an object 20 feet away; the patient's head was observed tilted slightly in the direction opposite the preferred eye and turned slightly in the direction of the preferred eye when the refractive status was symmetrical. That is, the patient with a symmetrical refractive status and right eye preferred was observed to tilt his head to the left and turn to the right. However, this was not necessarily the case when bilateral refractive status asymmetries, such as anisometropia, astigmatism, amblyopia, and strabismus were present.

This section focuses on anisometropia, amblyopia, and the related postural alterations.

A general statement can be made that asymmetric refractive conditions are a reflection of postural asymmetries. However, it cannot be demonstrated that all postural asymmetries are revealed in the refractive status.

"Asymmetric refractive conditions are a reflection of postural asymmetries."

The previously cited study revealed head turn in the direction equivalent to the eye with the greater refractive "error" in cases other than amblyopia. (Note: the term "error" is deliberately used here.) This was noted whether the condition was myopia, hyperopia or antimetropia.

Additional clinical observation conducted since the original study further evidences this principle. The eye on the side equivalent to the direction of turn is further away than the other eye from the viewed object. This may be a function of preferred eye; it is common (but not always) in myopia that the more myopic eye will be the preferred eye if there is anisometropia.

Perhaps a relationship exists between preferred eye and preferred side. The preferred side leads the way along the avenue of adaptation. This might explain the difference in postural adaptation observed in cases of amblyopia in which the opposite adaptation is revealed. When amblyopia exists, the direction of head turn is to the side opposite the amblyopic side. The final result is that the amblyopic eye is closer to the viewed object.

The following chart summarizes:

Condition	OD	OS	Head Turn	Eyes Turn
Myopia	More Less	Less More	Right Left	Left Right
Hyperopia	More Less	Less More	Right Left	Left Right
Antimetropia	More Less	Less More	Right Left	Left Right
Amblyopia	Amblyopic Normal	Normal Amblyopic	Left Right	Right Left

Editors note: "More" refers to the greater lens power in absolute value terms from plano. "Less" refers to the smaller lens power in absolute value terms from plano. Ex 1: OD –6.00 OS –2.00; the OD is More and the OS is Less. Ex 2: OD +5.00 OS +2.00; the OD is More and the OS is Less. Ex 3: OD +5.00 OS –2.00; the OD is More and the OS is Less.

Recall from the earlier parts of this chapter that the eyes turn in the direction opposite the direction of the pelvis' rotation. This can be stated quite differently; that is, the head turns in the direction of the rotation of the pelvis—the result being that the eyes turn in the opposite direction. In fact, this is a much more appropriate way to state this principle. All principles related to the influence, value and directives of the utilization of yoked prisms are derived from this insight.

Case studies of patients who illustrate the utilization of yoked prisms incorporated within the prescription as a therapeutic process were presented earlier in this chapter. Emphasis was placed on the Polaroid stereo tests to indicate the potential value and the direction of the bases of the prisms to be used. Recall the earlier statement, "Currently, Polaroid stereo tests provide the best indicators for the use of yoked prisms in lens prescribing, when the total optometric examination suggests the possibility."

The critical phrase in this statement is "when the total optometric examination suggests the possibility." The Polaroid stereo tests may "provide the best" indicator for yoked prisms to be used; but from a practical point of view, i.e., time, the examiner cannot be expected to probe every patient with various combinations of yoked prisms and note the effect on the Polaroid tests. Thus, one should probe "when the total optometric examination suggests the possibility." This possibility is suggested in three areas during the total optometric examination: head position observation, #15B (phoria through the fused cross cylinder) measurement, and refractive status.

The general rule shall be that the Polaroid stereo tests should be probed when one or more of these areas suggest the possibility. The following is a more detailed discussion of each area. Additionally, two visual training procedures that may suggest further probing with yoked prisms are discussed.

Head Position Observation

With the patient's attention fixated on an object across the room, such as the 20/200 letter, observe the position of the head turn. The possibility of yoked prisms' benefit is suggested when the head is turned in the direction opposite the preferred eye, or the head is turned exaggeratedly in the direction of the preferred eye.

#15B Measurement (phoria through the fused cross cylinder at near)

Earlier the author's standard procedure for doing the #15B test routinely was presented, as well as the variation performed on all phoria measurements of the analytical when anisometropia or antimetropia is revealed. To review, the target for #15B is a vertical column of reduced 20/20 letters on a nearpoint card placed at 16 inches (13 inches for children younger than 13 years). Dissociation prisms are introduced with total illumination. As a result, the patient is aware of two vertical columns of letters. The patient is instructed to read the letter on one of the targets and to report when the two columns of letters are in vertical alignment.

The variation introduced by the author is that the #15B finding is done twice—once reading the right eye's target and again reading the left eye's target. This is recorded as a right phoria and a left phoria. The right phoria is measured when reading the column of letters associated with the right eye, and the left phoria is measured when reading the column of letters associated with the left eye. If the difference between the two measurements is two prism diopters or greater, the possibility of the utilization of lateral yoked prisms exists and appropriate probing, using the Polaroid stereo tests, is indicated.

Earlier it was suggested that right and left phorias are taken on phoria tests and recorded when the refractive status reveals the asymmetry of anisometropia and antimetropia. Also, the same is true when the head position observations described above suggest asymmetric possibilities.

Refractive Status

The following guidelines related to the refractive status (#4 (retinoscopy), #5 (retinoscopy at 20 inches), #7 (subjective), #14A (unfused cross cylinder), and #14B (fused cross cylinder)) suggest appropriate yoked prism probing:

1. When one or more measures of refractive status reveal 0.50 diopter or more of anisometropia or antimetropia.
2. When any condition of myopia or adverse hyperopia is revealed in the #7 (subjective) finding. If the finding is symmetrical, probe with bases-up and bases-down yoked prisms. If the finding is asymmetrical (i.e., anisometropia or antimetropia), probe with all four bases (-up, -down, -right, and -left). If lateral yoked prisms, as well as vertical yoked prisms, are indicated as valuable, the following guidelines are suggested:
   a. Chances are great that lateral yoked prisms would be the ones of choice.
   b. On the other hand, begin with appropriate vertical yoked prisms unless there is some other indication as to prism base direction, if the vertical yoked prisms reveal greater improvement and/or decrement as compared to the lateral.
   c. Conceivably, there may be value in the use of obliquely oriented bases in these situations; the direction of the bases would be the vector resultant of the combinations. (This author has not done this or even investigated this possibility.) Hopefully, this will encourage some readers to initiate and ultimately report on such an investigation.
3. When amblyopia exanopsia is revealed.

"Not all postural asymmetry is revealed in the refractive status."

Previously the author noted that all asymmetric refractive conditions are reflections of postural asymmetry. However, not all postural asymmetry is revealed in the refractive status. Thus, it could be argued that the opportunity to probe the potential benefits gained from the utilization of yoked prisms should be provided routinely to all patients. Ultimately, this may be the case; certainly, it has not been the rule for this author. Time is always a factor; but, the need to probe, when indicated, outweighs the time factor. However, this author does not probe when the foregoing guidelines are not present.

Not all postural asymmetries are revealed in the optometric examination. Some patients accepted by this author for visual training have revealed postural asymmetries although such asymmetries were not disclosed during the examination. These postural asymmetries, in turn, reveal the value of lateral yoked prisms despite the fact that the patients had symmetrical refractive status and were not probed in the routine initial optometric examinations. This important information was learned as a result of the author's personal involvement in formalized visual training as part of a general optometric practice.

Motor Equivalence

The visual training procedure which best indicates this potential need for lateral yoked prisms is the activity known as motor equivalence. The basic motor equivalence procedure is for the patient to stand in front of a chalkboard with a piece of chalk held properly in each hand. The patient stands with feet slightly apart and weight equally distributed, facing a drawn X placed at eye level on the chalkboard. The chalk pieces are placed equally distant on either side of the fixated target (the X). While fixating on the X, the patient draws free and easy circles in opposite directions simultaneously with both hands and arms.

Possibly, lateral yoked prisms would be required as a training lens to be used for certain activities if the drawn circles are of unequal size. Lateral yoked prisms would be incorporated also in training lenses to be used at home and for near-centered activity. If the circles are asymmetric in size, the procedure is repeated with the patient standing on a balance board. Lateral yoked prisms are not indicated if the circles become equivalent in size under this condition. However, lateral yoked prisms probing is indicated (and the likelihood of their value is great) if the circles remain different sizes or become more exaggerated.

This procedure is repeated once again with the patient off the balance board. Again, he stands directly on the floor with feet apart and weight equally distributed. Lateral yoked prisms are worn; the procedure is repeated with bases-right yoked prisms first, and then second with bases-left. Obviously, it makes no difference which base direction is used first. The results are observed. One prism set will reduce the asymmetry. The other either may have no effect or further exaggerate the difference. The latter are the prisms to be used and incorporated as suggested above. Interestingly enough, lateral yoked prisms are NEVER used with the motor equivalence procedure for visual training purposes, but they are used with many other activities.

Lowman Tilted Balance Board

In addition to its visual training value, the Lowman Tilted Balance Board is another probe procedure customarily utilized in visual training which is useful to determine and confirm the value and base direction of lateral yoked prisms. When lateral yoked prisms are indicated as a value in visual training and, perhaps, as a value in general, the patient will be able to walk the balance board more easily with the appropriate yoked prism base direction. Walking with the inappropriate base direction will be more difficult and disturbing, and it will distort posture. The reader is referred to *Visual Training in Action* (written by this author and published by the Optometric Extension Program Foundation) for additional details on the motor equivalence procedure and the Lowman Tilted Balance Board.

The previous two examples further illustrate the possibility of adding these two activities to the routine complete optometric examination. My argument—at this time—against including the two activities would be, as already mentioned, the consideration of time. But this author will not say NEVER. Many things and/or routines may change as we learn more about behavioral aspects of optometry as well as appreciate all their potential applications.

Additional Prism Activity Considerations

Since formalized visual training examples have been discussed in this chapter, let us pursue the area of visual training a bit more. The chances are great that many clinicians—without even a realization or an appreciation—have used procedures with special lenses involving the postural alterations associated with the principles of yoked prisms. However, it is extremely important to appreciate the following considerations because better advantage of yoked prisms may be taken and there may be a time when what is done should be avoided.

Whenever prisms are used under monocular conditions or dissociated conditions, the resultant behavior is identical to that occurring when yoked prisms are used routinely. For example, when monocular base-in prism is used (as it was recommended years ago) in conjunction with a given procedure, i.e., one eye occluded, the resulting postural response is the same as with lateral yoked bases-left prisms as long as the monocular prism base-in was before the right eye. Also, the postural response is identical to that occurring when using a pair of bases-up yoked prisms when the target fixated is that associated with the base-up eye under dissociated conditions using, for example, vertical prisms (base-up before one eye, base-down before the other). Obviously the converse is true.

The response is identical to that associated with base-left prisms when dissociating prism base-in is worn and when the patient views the right eye's target. Again, the converse is true. Thus, the reader can interpolate what the case would be if dissociating base-out prisms are worn.

Finally, the strabismic should be considered briefly. It was not unusual for many years to include prism (frequently small degrees of base-in with the prescription for a convergent strabismic) in a visual training program. More recently, Israel Greenwald, O.D., has encouraged the use of over-compensating prism (base-out) in similar cases.

Perhaps if there is any value in the use of such prisms (either base direction), it may lie in the value of the postural response, which results from viewing through conditions identical to those associated with yoked prisms.

CHAPTER 10
The Behavioral Concept and Patient Management

The earlier parts of this book have been concerned primarily with the clinical application of lenses related to and derived from theoretical concepts associated with behavioral aspects of optometry.

Much has been said regarding the utilization of lenses for purposes other than compensation—the conventional wisdom approach. The determination and value of lenses, spheres and yoked prisms have been described for purposes of prevention, protection, control, maintenance and improvement of visual performance. These lenses have been called counter-stress or stress-relieving lenses. It has been noted, implied and stated precisely that the specific dioptric values of such lenses are not among the findings of the analytical examination. The value of such lenses to the patient, however, is derived as a product of behavioral considerations in the optometric analysis of the analytical examination data.

The word value has been used in association with lenses, both "dioptric value" and "patient value." As a noun, the word value means "that which renders anything desirable or useful;" however, the verb value is defined as "to estimate the worth of." It is appropriate to shift our attention temporarily from the use of value as a noun to its use as a verb. It is time to consider the word *value* in terms of dollars.

In the final analysis the optometrist must put a dollar sign on a proposed program of optometric care and the patient must view the benefits of the program in relation to the proposed fee.

This brings us to a most important topic—practice management as it relates to the behavioral concept.

Selling is inherent in practice management. An optometrist has the most important commodity to sell his patients, the commodity of VISION. From vision, meaning is derived and action is directed. The value of compensatory lens care alone is significant to the patient. Consequently, then, how valuable can prevention, protection, control, maintenance and/or improvement of vision and visual performance be to a patient? Only an individual optometrist can answer this question in terms of dollars. Despite great knowledge of theoretical concepts and extremely capable clinical know-how, if an optometrist lacks patient management skills, patients will suffer. A successful practice, both for the optometrist and patients must integrate concept insight, clinical capability and practice management. If an optometrist is not successful financially, then it is impossible to provide benefits, which lead to enthusiastic, excited and successful patients.

"People buy the benefits of a product if they are significant."

Patient management is a function of practice management. Another label for patient management is selling. Like other professionals, the optometrist is a professional salesman with a most important commodity to sell—vision. In reality the optometrist sells and the patient buys. But what does the patient buy? What motivates the patient to buy?

The answers to these two questions are the essence of this chapter as well as the true significance of a behavioral approach to optometry.

Some may object to the use of common marketplace terms like selling and buying. Nevertheless, the words are accurate. Selling vision is providing vision care and this is optometry. The patient buys what the optometrist sells. What motivates a patient to buy and pay the required fee relates to projected and predicted benefits, which a patient can derive as a product of purchase.

People buy the benefits of a product if they are significant. The more they appreciate the significance, the easier it is both to sell and to buy. This is as true in professional activities as in the business world. If benefits satisfy needs, then people buy; and they are satisfied when the anticipated benefits are derived. On the other hand, if benefits are greater than initially anticipated, then people not only are satisfied, they are also enthusiastic. The professional optometric goal should always be an enthusiastic patient. The application of the behavioral concept provides this opportunity more than any other clinical optometric approach. This author's practice is oriented totally to this goal.

This author graduated from Pennsylvania College of Optometry and shortly thereafter began the development of a general full-scope practice of optometry, which included formalized visual training as only one area of the practice—not as a specialty. Early on the author realized that a successful general practice depended on many factors.

A few of these factors are:

1. Development of a practice population desiring to being programmed for optometric care throughout their life
2. Development of enthusiastic patients

3. A referral source for new patients primarily being other patients instead of professional referrals
4. Cultivating the concept of being the family optometrist

"Enthusiastic patients are those who derive more benefits than they initially expect."

Satisfied patients are those who have successfully derived what they expected; unless they are enlightened to the behavioral concept, their care usually meant application of a viewpoint other than the behavioral concept. In other words, they were provided minimum level vision care. On the other hand, as stated earlier, enthusiastic patients are those who derive more and greater benefits than what they initially expect.

Enthusiastic patients are the greatest referral source. They want to share with their family and friends the benefits they have derived. They refer.

Once "the word is out," it is not unusual for optometrists and non-optometrists to refer new patients because of the benefits derived as a product of the behavioral concept, particularly where visual training is concerned.

Yet many years ago, the author learned that, for the proper development and maintenance of a desired type of practice, it was unwise to permit excessive non-patient new patient referrals. He found such a policy to be not only unwise, but also inconsistent with his goals. Therefore, he has limited the professional referral of new patients to 10%. For example, 90% of all new patients are derived from patient referral.

The author recalls once when an enthusiastic patient, who was a pediatrician, wanted him to see all of his patients! He agreed to see only a maximum of 10 of this pediatrician's patients per year—his choice—no more. Unquestionably, the enthusiastic patient is an optometrist's best pubic relations agent.

"The enthusiastic patient is an optometrist's best public relations agent"

A new patient (and in the case of a child, the parent) knows at least two major facts about the author's office before visiting. (We make sure a new patient knows these.) They are as follows:

1. The complete diagnostic optometric examination and evaluation requires a minimum of two office visits. The first office visit is for the examination. Assuming the total investigation can be completed in one visit, the patient (and/or parents in case of a child) returns for a second office visit for the evaluation conference. The first office visit takes a maximum of one hour. The second visit is one-half hour.

2. There is a minimum fee to come into the office. This fee entitles the patient to a diagnostic examination and evaluation. We always use the term "minimum" fee because the "entrance" fee will be more than the minimum if a diagnostic examination requires additional office visits.

The "entrance" fee is exactly what it implies. It is an entrance fee that creates the possibility of significant initial benefits and the opportunity for a lifelong program of vision care designed to prevent, protect, control, maintain and improve visual performance as determined by the needs and desires of the patient. It is not an "examination" fee. The author does not condone such a concept; he has no such fee. The reader may appreciate later, if not already, that charging a fee for an examination is inconsistent and incompatible with the practice management aspects of this author's application of behavioral concepts.

The vast majority of new patients require only the minimum two office-visit procedure. Only rarely is the second supplementary office visit needed for further examination. A review of case studies reported in previous chapters reveals what is done during the first office visit. There are three essential aspects:

1. Patient history
2. Eye health screening
3. Optometric investigation of vision (visual abilities, visual performance, and vision function) by means of:
   a. The analytical examination
   b. Visual performance tests

Prior to the patient's (and/or parents') return for the evaluation conference appointment, the author takes the necessary time to analyze, appraise and evaluate the collected data to derive recommendations. The reader may have the following questions: "Why is it necessary to bring the patient into the office for an additional visit?" "Why not proceed immediately after the examination with the discussion?" The author is frequently asked these questions by other optometrists, questions that relate to the patient's willingness to return for such a conference.

Let's answer these questions in reverse order. There is never a question or reluctance in the patient's mind in returning for this second visit. This routine is understood in advance as being standard operating procedure for this office. It is also understood that the conference is crucial to the patient's welfare. The author learned long ago that the need for this second visit was essential to understand all of the insights and implications derived from the examination and to communicate these along with appropriate recommendations in the shortest time possible.

Another long-established principle involved in the "art of selling" is that the salesman—in this instance, the optometrist—simultaneously must be highly organized, well rehearsed, fresh and spontaneous. Marguerite T. Eberl, O.D., a famous optometrist, once said, "My most spontaneous remarks are very carefully rehearsed." Rest assured that this author's spontaneous remarks are always carefully rehearsed!

The primary purpose or goal of the conference appointment is to convey insight and information to the patient relative to his vision status, recognition of the patient's needs and any recommendations, which could satisfy those needs. The conference also has secondary goals and purposes related to information, which is peripheral to the patient, yet essential for the patient to appreciate. The patient must have the opportunity to select and be measured for his frame, if glasses are required, within the half-hour structure of this conference. There is much to be done in a relatively short period of time in the most expedient and comprehensive way possible. This requires organization, structure and rehearsal.

The optometrist also should remain in control, and proper preparation provides this opportunity. This, then, is an opportunity for significant benefits not only for this patient, but also for all the potential patients he will refer as an enthusiastic patient. Preparation time also provides an opportunity for the clinician to review the type of patient or parents to whom he will communicate. The clinician can then prepare the most effective language for communication. The reader is referred for more details on this point to "Communicating for Success," an important course authored by Harold Wiener, O.D., and published by the Optometric Extension Program.[1]

In addition to assuring the patient that the eye health screening did not reveal evidence of ocular pathology (assuming that this is correct), A.M. Skeffington, O.D. (the late Director of Education of OEP) always said that there were four primary questions in the patient's mind to answer. The answers to these questions comprise the primary purposes and goals of the conference. The four questions are:

1. "Do I have a visual problem?"
2. "Do I have a visual problem you can help me solve?"
3. "How much does it cost?"
4. "How do I pay for it?"

An important aspect of the primary goal is that the patient is given insight as to why his symptoms, as expressed in terms of need, are related to an inadequacy in visual functioning and visual performance. The patient requires some degree of physiological justification. Obvious inadequacies noted by the patient during the investigation of visual performance should be reviewed. One example is suppression as seen on the Telebinocular.

The secondary goal and purpose of the conference is to give the patient greater insight and understanding of vision and the types of vision care, which may be significant, both to him and others he may refer. The patient should understand that visual dysfunction is the result of a thwarting in development and/or stress-induced as a product of responding to the stressor-agent of biologically unacceptable, socially compulsive, visually near-centered demands.

Recognizing this, we are vitally and primarily interested in prevention. How wonderful it is when we see youngsters at an early age and when we can help prevent visual problems and dysfunction. And even if visual dysfunction already exists (therefore, too late to prevent), it is not too late to provide an opportunity to protect, control and maintain stability in visual functioning.

Finally, I believe it is important for every patient to appreciate that visual training can benefit everyone who has needs that cannot be satisfied by a simpler approach to vision care. If needed, every human being could learn to see more efficiently and effectively. A patient with such information and insight can play a significant role by informing others of his or her case; in so doing the patient helps respond to the visual needs of his or her family and/or friends. As your public relations agent, your patient can recognize when others should be referred to you.

The analysis, evaluation and appraisal of data and information collected during the examination office visit lead to conclusions and recommendations for the patient in relationship to the patient's symptoms and needs.

The four basic questions in the patient's mind can be answered adequately during the evaluation conference appointment. The steps involved during the preparation time related to the analysis, evaluation, and appraisal are the following:

1. The Skeffington Analytical Sequence of case analysis is applied. The data of the analytical examination (21-point examination) is checked, chained and typed. The resultant is subjected to the seven Directives of Lens Application from which is derived a prescribable lens formula. Today, this is frequently referred to as the safe lens prescription, which actually means that it is a prescription for glasses that the optometrist can feel assured that the patient will wear (and never was intended for

any other purpose). In no way does it imply that it is the optimum or best lens prescription or the best and only approach to vision care. In order to use the analytical examination data for this purpose, it is essential that the individual measurements of the analytical be done precisely as described in the "Little Black Book," which is available from the OEP. (The Behavioral Optometry Approach to Lens Prescribing, Homer Hendrickson, O.D., Revised Edition). If this is not done, the data are not reliable or usable in the manner for which the analytical was designed.

2. The status of adaptation is appraised. The appropriate data of the analytical examination, which relate to the degree of embeddedness or non-embeddedness, is analyzed and conclusions are drawn as to the status. The behavior may be non-embedded, partially embedded or embedded.

3. All the optometric examination data, including history, are evaluated and appraised as to the status of adaptation, the etiology, the symptoms and the expressed needs. The data reveal the nature of current visual performance and the resulting manifestations of dysfunction and conditions. These relate to the symptoms and expressed needs. It is important to have some insight into the patient's total behavior, how it is expressed, what the patient has done in terms of adaptation, and to have some appreciation as to its origin. Is the behavior an expression of a vision development problem, a stress-induced dysfunction or a combination? Does the behavior reveal a primary stress-induced visual problem in addition to what is now revealed as a secondary condition? Is an adaptation revealed which requires compensatory lenses to satisfy certain needs in addition to appropriate counter-stress lenses? How did performance change or behavior alter with the introduction of probe lenses? Answers to these questions provide for the ultimate understanding of the patient's visual behavior, performance and needs. Previously, reference was made to the patient's four questions, which need to be answered. Likewise, the optometrist must have four questions in his own mind, which must be answered. These questions can be answered after proceeding with the prior analytical processing; it is essential to answer the questions before attempting to answer the patient's questions. These four questions are as follows:
   a. Does the patient have a visual problem?
   b. Does the patient have a visual problem that I can help him solve, and, if so, how?
   c. Is a team approach required?
   d. If so, who should be the captain of the team?

4. The results of this analysis are prepared in written outline form—primarily for the benefit of the author—to be used as organized notes to report to the patient at the conference. Actually, a copy of these prepared notes is made for the patient (see Appendix A).

There are at least five reasons for this. First, it permits the patient to listen and communicate during the conference and to raise questions and to interact instead of feeling compelled to hang on every word said and/or to take notes. Second, it ensures that the patient leaves the office with a written summary for future reference of his visual condition, written recommendations and associated fees. Having such a copy leaves nothing to chance. Third, the patient is free to make copies and distribute them as desired, if he wishes to use these notes as a report. We do not and will not write reports. Fourth, it serves as excellent public relations. And fifth, it is a good souvenir, if nothing else.

These notes are constructed in two parts. Part one is comprised of a series of specifics in numerical order gleaned from the examination.

The number one statement in part one is an abbreviated statement of the vision condition and etiology, such as an "embedded stress-induced visual problem, reduced visual efficiency." The number two statement always relates to the health status of the eye; for example, the investigation for ocular pathology and abnormality was negative. Then follow—point-by-point—salient facts, symptoms, and complaints reported by the patient during the history. Next, the significant observations revealed during the course of the optometric examination are reported point by point. Finally, there is a summation statement on the condition and its significance to the patient, including his performance and behavior.

"All patients are provided with alternatives of optometric care."

Part two relates to the recommendations for the patient. All patients are provided with alternatives of optometric care placed under the heading, "Optometric Care Program Alternatives." As suggested earlier, selling is an art. People do not enjoy being dictated to; they also do not appreciate ultimatums. Choices are preferred. Any individual prefers the opportunity to select the alternative which best satisfies his needs. This is a truism in any aspect of life—behavior and sales.

Essentially, the behavioral concept in optometry provides an opportunity to offer any patient alternatives of optometric care. Each alternative of care provides a certain level of benefits varying in the order of good, better and best. The patient will have the opportunity to balance the benefits gained from each alternative against his desires and needs and cost. Then, the patient determines the level of care he wants. Thus, the patient plays the proper role of decision maker, and the optometrist plays his proper role determining the nature of the condition and the reason for the patient's behavior and he has provided the patient with various approaches.

Alternatives of Care

The three alternatives derived from the evaluation are as follows:

A. Conventional care (good)
B. Functional care (better)
C. Visual training (best)

For all practical purposes, the behavioral concept will permit the derivation of these alternatives for everyone. Conventional care, the first alternative, is the recommendation of the lens formula (which could be no prescription) as derived from the OEP method of case analysis. Essentially, this is the level of care a patient might expect or get from any vision care clinician. If a lens formula is revealed, the patient can be expected to attain from it a certain level of predictable benefit. There are some patients who desire only this level of care. When it is time to discuss the alternatives of care in the course of the conference, this author's opening gambit related to the conventional level is the following: "If all I know today is what was known or done in our field two and one-half to three generations ago, this is all I would be able to offer you." This is of particular significance to the parents of a youngster with a learning-related visual problem, who has 20/20, healthy eyes, no ocular defects, and no lens formula prescribable, yet who has had prior vision examination and been told there was "nothing wrong."

The functional care alternative indicates the uniqueness of the behavioral concept and the power of lenses. This alternative provides for lenses directed toward prevention, protection, control, maintenance and/or improvement of visual performance. This level of care is the subject of this book. It is one thing to be able to determine the availability of lens power to alter behavior in the course of the examination; but one can be firm in his or her convictions and predict and determine the benefits to be attained by means of such lenses only as a result of the total analysis inherent in the behavioral concept. It is standard procedure to program the patient for an initial progress case study following use of such lenses at a specific time one to three months following utilization. Then, future programming is determined.

Visual training (VT) is the third alternative and is offered to everyone. This alternative recognizes that every human being can develop a more efficient and effective visual system; however, not everyone has needs and/or desires, which require visual training. If nothing else, this serves to provide valuable information to any patient as to the availability of visual training and its potential benefits for others and himself. Frequently, a patient may realize that he wants to take advantage of the opportunity when the potential benefits to be gained by visual training exceed the benefits provided by means of the other alternatives.

Given the opportunity to select among alternatives of good, better and best, the distribution of sales is consistent—about 10% purchase good, 70% better, and 20% best. Ironically, the percentage breakdown of the author's patients "buying" the alternatives is identical over the many years of providing patients with three alternatives of vision care. Given the opportunity, the vast majority of patients desire a level of care beyond minimum level care to which they have so often been subjected as the only approach.

Fees for Benefits

It was stated earlier that people buy benefits derived from vision care provided by the optometrist. People buy benefits no matter what the commodity. The fee is acceptable if the benefits to be gained are within their abilities to pay. The discussion of fees, the determination of fees and the principles related to the fee always are very difficult to consider; but this is a necessity of life and reality.

It is not uncommon for a patient to be charged a specific amount for an examination plus a fee for glasses, as determined by the costs of frame and lenses. In this author's practice, the patient cannot "buy" an examination. There is no examination fee. The patient cannot even "buy" a pair of glasses. Although we provide glasses, we do not sell glasses. The only commodities a patient can "buy" in this author's practice are benefits. This begins with the initial entrance fee.

A fee is predetermined for each alternative and is recorded on the outline. The fee is commensurate with the benefits to be gained and will vary according to the potential benefits. The more benefit to be gained, the higher the fee. Visual training fees are pre-established and standardized. The fees vary only with the approach and the nature of the program (They will not be discussed at length in this book.). Additionally, the entrance fee is absorbed within the total fee for either the first or second alternative.

It should be emphasized (and rather obvious) that this author disagrees with a prior existing concept of fees in which the patient pays for time, skill and knowledge of the clinician. This sounded good and it seemed super professional—at least it was made to appear so. Once again, however, the bottom line is that people are willing to pay only for benefits. They could care less about one's time, skill and knowledge.

The first alternative, the conventional minimum level vision care approach fee, will be significantly less than the second alternative. Minimum fees are influenced by standard office procedure, i.e., chair cost, costs of materials and the desired minimum level of income. The add-on for the second alternative is determined by benefit levels likely to be attained by the patient. The actual total figure must be determined within the mind of the optometrist, who asks himself the question: "What are these benefits worth?" As an example, the more non-embedded the behavior, the more benefits that can be anticipated. Thus, it can be expected that the fee for the second alternative in the non-embedded patient will be significantly greater than that for the similar patient whose behavior is more embedded.

At this point, the significance of the second alternative as contrasted with the first alternative should be obvious. Case studies considered in preceding chapters demonstrated this significance as well as potential benefits to patients. Recognizing that at least 70% of people want the benefits of the second alternative as contrasted with the first alternative, given the opportunity, the difference in the optometrist's income should, likewise, be obvious.

It was stated earlier in this chapter that this author provides glasses to the patient, but that a patient cannot buy a pair of glasses. Again, the principle relates to the fact that patients buy benefits to be gained. Actually, the office buys the glasses from the laboratory and gives the glasses to the patient. The glasses are the means to an end, not the end product. The glasses are not the commodity; the benefits to be gained are the commodity.

"The fee paid is for the program of optometric care, not glasses."

Therefore, when the alternatives are discussed along with the fees at the conference, the patient is informed that he or she will select a frame of his or her choice and the office will buy the patient a pair of glasses and supply him or her with such ophthalmic materials no matter which alternative is selected. The fee paid is for the program of optometric care, not glasses.

Periodically, a patient asks whether he or she can take a copy of his or her prescription to get it filled. Perhaps the patient has a friend or relative in the optical business or maybe is aware of the periodic advertising of glasses. This author has no objection to this. However, it is ridiculous for patients to spend additional money for glasses when they are going to be given a pair of glasses at no cost—that is, unless they desire a second pair. Again, understand that the fee is for the program of care and it is not varied or reduced if the patient has additional glasses procured outside the office. The patient cannot get glasses for less money from someone else because in our office the glasses are given to him or her; they are not sold to the patient.

It is also important to know in these days of insured health care that the second alternative—with the exception of pure preventive lens utilization—is considered optometric visual training. It is covered by those health care plans that cover visual training.

Let us now return to the evaluation and preparation time prior to the patient's return for the conference. It is important to report that it takes an average of 15 minutes per patient to analyze, evaluate and write an outline for the conference.

"The patient...buys an opportunity of lifelong vision care."

In the language of selling, the purpose of the conference is to sell a program of optometric care. The patient buys a program of optometric care equivalent to his level of need and expected benefits. At that time the sale is closed. If the patient selects an alternative other than the first, he also buys an opportunity of lifelong vision care associated with the benefits derived from the behavioral concept, i.e., prevention, protection, control, maintenance and/or improvement of visual performance. This is an option, and it is the patient's opportunity to avail himself of this care and, if so desired, the patient will be programmed appropriately. If the first alternative is selected, the patient obviously is not interested in the higher level of benefits. Actually, he could have derived this level of service at even the minimum of vision care services available. This patient denies himself the opportunity and option provided to others. As in days of old, it is as though, "Here's a pair of glasses to satisfy your needs; come back and see me when you feel the need," or "If you so desire, we will program you to reevaluate your status in one year."

Obviously, anyone selecting the third alternative, visual training, will resort—when completed—to the programming of vision care associated with the programming and control of the second-alternative patient. Thus, the patient will have the opportunity and the option to reap all the future rewards of programmed vision care.

The initial reevaluation examination progress case study with the second alternative is included as part of the services provided. The initial case study is not completed until the patient returns for this office visit. Additional data is collected at that time and the ensuing behavior is appraised.

Then, future programming is determined based on the responses and behavior revealed. This future programming is consistent with the best interests of the patient in association with the behavioral concept. For example, the patient may be programmed to return in one year for an annual complete reevaluation examination or it may be desirable to see the patient again for a progress case study in three or six months—whatever is best. If additional glasses or a change in lenses is required, these will be supplied either at our "processing cost" to the patient or, if desired, the patient may have the prescription to fill somewhere else. This is acceptable to the author as long as the patient agrees to return with such materials for our approval. The annual complete reevaluation examination appointment requires a 45-minute period of time. The shorter progress case studies are scheduled for one-half hour.

Again, there is no "examination" fee; but the patient pays an office visit fee for all appointments other than the initial progress case study included as part of the second alternative.

Annual programming of reevaluation examination appointments are controlled. Patients request that they be called one month in advance of the due month by the office and an appointment is arranged. The progress case studies are controlled by prearranging the appointment and sending the patient a notice of the appointment date and time. Obviously, the office reconfirms all appointments by phone the day before.

A sample copy of a conference outline form is included for further reference as part of this chapter (see Appendix A). The next section will provide additional elaboration of the principles set forth in this chapter.

Stress and programmed vision care

This chapter has discussed and described patient management in the context of a behavioral approach to optometric care. With the assumption that the patient desires the level of benefit that can be afforded and is unique to such a practice, the optometrist's goal is to provide the patient the opportunity of programmed vision care throughout life. The purpose of such care is to prevent vision dysfunction and visual problems as well as provide the opportunity to protect, control and maintain visual performance and visual abilities. In addition, enhancement of visual performance and visual abilities are provided whenever necessary and desired.

The purpose of programmed vision care in the behavioral approach to optometric practice is summed up well in the following hypothetical monologue in which the optometrist and the patient are at the conclusion of the progress case study. This progress case study was part of the original optometric care program providing the level of benefit desired by the patient and predicted by the optometrist:

> *You have demonstrated and proven to me that you have attained the benefits you desired and now it's your job to maintain these benefits, and our obligation to see to it that you do maintain them. If it is at all possible, we never want to see you again when you have developed visual problems—we want to keep you free of problems, and throughout the coming years, we are going to do our part to fulfill this obligation to you. In order to do this, we want to see you next for an annual complete vision examination, not for one of these progress case studies, but for a complete examination, similar to our original, in one year. This is the next step in our program to help you maintain your present level of visual abilities throughout life.*
>
> *Do understand that we want to prevent your having additional visual problems: we're not going to wait for you to have more problems. We would not think very much of a dentist who said, 'Now, your teeth are in fine shape; when they start bothering you again, let me hear from you and we'll fill them again.' And, likewise and, more importantly, the same is true with your vision and visual abilities.*
>
> *You can't afford to lose what you now have. And, since numerous factors can enter into your life, such as a change in the demands of your job, or even normal physiological changes, which are stressful and can interfere with your visual abilities, we're going to see you periodically to reevaluate your abilities, and make sure that you always have the proper protecting lenses. At present, I would predict that you will be using this current prescription of lenses probably for a few years, but I'm not interested in seeing you for the purpose of changing your glasses. In fact, undoubtedly, there will be prescriptive changes over the years as you follow through with this program, but I hope that you will never be AWARE of the need for the lens change, because if you are, it's too late to prevent. The very fact that you are aware of a need is an indication that you are in trouble. The periodic programmed examination will reveal if and when lens changes are required rather than your awareness. Our responsibility is to keep you free of problems.*
>
> *Therefore, we'll plan to see you next in one year. This will give us a control in terms of time. And for your convenience, if you would like, we shall have the secretary call you one month prior to the month you are due, and she will arrange the appointment for you.*

Programmed Vision Care

Each new patient has the potential opportunity for programmed vision care, which begins the moment the initial request for the optometric examination appointment is made. It is an option, not a requirement. The patient or parent has the opportunity to explore this option. A patient who chooses conventional level vision care as an alternative implies that minimum level vision care provides benefits that satisfy his needs. This patient is satisfied with the level of care equated with the dentist who filled his cavities—he will return only when his teeth have additional decay.

"The behavioral optometrist can only deal totally with a certain number of patients, determined and limited by the number of hours per year available in the examining room."

The foregoing hypothetical conversation is suggestive of the nature of discussion held with patients who have selected levels of a behavioral approach to optometric care and have reaped the initial benefits. At the time of such discussion, all patients do agree and request that they be called for the annual programmed examination. They have taken the initial step in accepting their option for programmed vision care. One year later they will have the opportunity to again accept or deny themselves this opportunity when the phone call is received for arranging the appointment. If they do not arrange for the appointment, obviously they have denied themselves the opportunity, at this time, for programmed vision care. This is their decision. A patient may decide against further vision care for many reasons, including a lack of understanding of the long-range benefits. Although this rarely occurs, it is either the problem of the optometrist in failing to communicate initially or simply that the patient no longer cares—this author is convinced that the usual reason is the former. Interestingly enough, the author's practice reveals about an 80% positive response to patients offered the opportunity of programmed vision care. This, of course, demonstrates and implies another advantage of the behavioral approach in an optometric practice in that it is not dependent upon volume of patients. The optometrist can only deal totally with a certain number of patients, determined and limited by the number of hours per year available in the examining room. The approximate 10% conventional level care patients automatically deny themselves programmed care. The small percentage of other patients denying themselves the same care permits and assures some appointment time being available for new patients.

If conditions were ideal, programmed vision care would begin with patients being seen, not because anything was wrong, but because everything was good and the desire was to keep it that way. Contrary to conventional care principles, ideally the patient begins his programmed vision care free of symptoms and identifiable vision disabilities. The patient's need and desire should be to do anything necessary to remain free of visual problems and vision conditions. This level of vision care may be sought by patients of any age. However, the chances are great that unless the patient is initially seen at early school age or, even better, during preschool ages, the programming of optometric care would be directed toward protecting, controlling and maintaining visual abilities rather than preventive vision care. Recall that most vision disabilities occur during the school-age years, and a much smaller percentage (vision development problems) arise during the preschool years. Remember that there is a difference between a visual problem and a vision condition.

Alternatives of Care

Assuming that the initial diagnostic examination and evaluation revealed no evidence of dysfunction or visual problem, alternatives of optometric care are presented. Alternative #1, or conventional level care, would be to do nothing, recommend nothing, and the patient would return if and when symptoms or needs arose. Alternative #3 is always visual training; but to be accepted for visual training requires that the patient's needs can be satisfied only by such a program—having needs implies and defines the existence of a visual problem. Such a patient as being discussed has no visual problem and, therefore, is not acceptable for visual training. Nevertheless, from a public relations point of view it is important to discuss this aspect.

Alternative #2, functional level care, will be vision care directed towards the prevention of vision disabilities and visual problems. At the preschool age this can involve providing information to parents about desirable activities and environmental factors, which support and encourage vision development. The parents are given insight related to factors, which can thwart development and, thus, should be avoided. The future is discussed in terms of the child's potential vulnerability to stress-related, near-centered demands. At such a time, preventive lenses will be recommended. If prevention is the goal, such lenses will be a necessity. Finally, unless indicated otherwise, the child is programmed to be seen again in one year for comparative analysis of vision, visual abilities and visual performance. This pattern of programming continues until vulnerability is revealed.

A patient older than preschool age who is free of visual problems and dysfunction, but is vulnerable, needs appropriate stress-relieving lenses for preventive purposes. If this level of care, Alternative #2, is desired and accepted, such lenses, generally in dual focus form with Plano uppers, are provided and the patient is instructed to use them for all near-centered activities. Programming of vision care is continued in that the patient will be seen again in one year. Here again lies the answer to the question asked of Skeffington, "Would you put lenses on every child?" Rather than dogmatically answering, "Yes," a better answer is to state that the patient is offered the opportunity of preventive vision care when the vulnerability is revealed. Ideally, the answer is "Yes," and if the importance of vision is appreciated, the inclination is acceptability of the proposed program of preventive vision care.

Two related factors must be considered. First, prevention is the hardest service to sell in any field or area, particularly in vision care when the primary preventive means is glasses. Second, both the optometrist and the patient (or parent) must understand that just because one is vulnerable, the optometrist cannot be sure as to when and if vision disability may arise. It is likely if one remains in the environment of the cultural demands that contribute to the emergence of such dysfunction, sooner or later such dysfunction will emerge in one form or another.

The optometrist must be prepared to cope with these factors when vulnerability is revealed and preventive care involving stress-relieving lenses is to be recommended. Relative to the above factors, the patient (or parent) may not accept the recommendation for preventive lenses. The optometrist should be appreciative of the emotion involved and approach this situation from a positive point of view. An alternative option exists that does not preclude the continuation of programmed vision care. It is a gamble if the patient does not use the stress-relieving lenses, but some people prefer to wait until the earliest evidence of response to stress is revealed. Recall that if the dysfunction is seen at the earliest stage, the non-embedded stage, the program of care primarily involves the use of counter-stress lenses for therapeutic purposes; when the dysfunction is alleviated, such lenses are continued for maintenance and preventive purposes. In these situations the programming of vision care continues with the patient being seen annually at the very least. Appropriate positive vision care steps are taken when evidence is revealed that satisfies the patient's or parents' emotional level of understanding. Then lenses are provided. When the vulnerability manifests itself, we come to a fork in the road. The alternatives are either to proceed immediately with preventive lenses or wait until first evidence of response is demonstrated—this is a patient's decision, not the optometrist's. The optometrist's obligation is to ensure that the patient or parent understands this. This author's experience suggests that, given the opportunity for preventive vision care, 65% take immediate advantage of the preventive lens approach when they are ready for them.

Rarely, a patient of young adult or adult age will be seen who reveals no visual problem, no vision condition and no evidence of vulnerability. Also rarely, a patient of a similar age level may be seen who exhibits no visual problem or vision dysfunction, but does reveal vulnerability. The former is the rarest occurrence. In 33 years of practice, this author has seen only four people from age 16 to 35 who revealed no evidence of vulnerability yet were very much involved with the near-centered demands of our culture. Interestingly, all four patients have been female with extremely high capabilities and acknowledged very high intelligence quotients, one of whom was in Harvard University at age 14. Obviously these patients have never been provided with stress-relieving lenses nor has such been recommended, but they have been continuously programmed for annual optometric examination to make sure all remains right. They are prepared for the time if and when they will need and profit from stress-relieving lenses. If nothing else, sooner or later the internal stress of presbyopia will be revealed and, at that time, appropriate counter-stress lenses have been or will be provided.

Preventive Vision Care Concepts

"...preventive vision care is unique to the behavioral concept of vision."

Throughout these chapters it has been both implied and stated specifically that the consideration and implementation of preventive vision care is unique to the behavioral concept of vision. No other concept of vision gives attention, concern or insight into prevention because either (1) the theory implies structural defects and is fatalistic or (2) there is no consideration of etiology, and thus the resultant observation of dysfunction is an existence with no concern regarding wherefrom or why it exists.

In addition, if visual disability is revealed, the primary concern, once again unique to a behavioral approach, has to do with protection, control and maintenance of existing visual abilities as well as remediation of dysfunction and enhancement of visual performance as may be needed, desired and required. Visual problems are products of either interference in development or interference on that which has been developed, the former being labeled vision development problems and the latter, stress-induced visual problems. Both clinical insight, as well as available data, reveal that the vast majority of vision conditions are those labeled stress-induced visual problems emerging in increasing incidence as the school-age years advance. Reference has continually been made to the behavioral utilization of lenses, referring to these lenses as counter-stress, or its synonym, stress-relieving. The implication is that these lenses serve to reduce, relieve or eliminate stress.

Three questions arise:

1. What is stress?
2. What is THE stress?
3. Where is stress?

The late Hans Selye, M.D., defined stress as the nonspecific response of the body to any demand made upon it.[2,3,4] He noted that stress was essential for life, and further differentiated between stress and the stressor-agent, the latter being that which produces stress. In other words, the stressor-agent is the demander and stress is a response within the body. That stress is not negative, not bad, is of utmost importance to appreciate. Behavior requires stress, which, in turn, is dependent upon stressor-agents to induce stress. Stress is more often constructive rather than adverse but it can be said, in general, that the response of the body to a demand made upon it is adaptation. This is adjustment and learning. The stressor-agent creates a problem to be solved; the solving of the problem is the response, the adaptation.

Identified dysfunction in the visual system is evidence of adverse adaptation to stress. The evidence of unimpaired visual performance reveals that that person is presently coping with the demands imposed upon it without the need of maladaptation.

As Selye stated, stress is essential for life, for behavior, for movement, for learning, for survival. Physiologically, the living organism is designed to meet and cope with stress. This is exactly what Harmon meant with his oft-quoted statement, "The organism grows along a line of stress to reduce stress."[5] As implied before, stress may be positive or negative, constructive or adverse, depending on the adaptation required. If the adaptation does not require bodily structure alteration, it is constructive, resulting in the solution of a problem, movement and learning. If change in structure is created in order to survive, the problem is solved but at an expense to the organism, and this is adverse adaptation or maladaptation and optometrically will be seen as vision dysfunction.

It can be further stated and clarified that the living organism is designed to meet transient stress without need of adverse adaptation but persisting stress does require bodily structural alteration and results in maladaptation. Persistency of stress involves both time and intensity. The greater the duration of the imposed stress and/or the degree of intensity of the demand, the greater the chance for a resulting persisting stress rather than a transient stress.

Induced stress requires increased energy demands, energy utilization and effort. The basic goal of the organism is to function with minimal effort and the least expenditure of energy. Thus, once again, when stress is produced, the organismic drive is to solve the problem and reduce the stress in order to perform with minimal expenditure on the part of the person. This is problem solving, adaptation and learning. The drive is to habituate the performance which is least energy demanding. If the stress is persisting, the person must adapt to find the means to reduce energy expenditure.

The socially compulsive, biologically unacceptable, near-centered demand is one example, and the most common example, of a stressor-agent resulting in visual dysfunction. This would be an example of a vision disability resulting from interference in the developed visual process, and is referred to in general as a stress-induced visual problem. Note, however, that near-centered activities are not the only stressor-agent inducing and resulting in the stress-induced visual problem. Additional stressor-agents related to both internal and external environmental forces can result in identical and similar syndromes. Years ago, this syndrome of vision dysfunction was referred to as a nearpoint visual problem, implying the etiology to be the use of the eyes for near vision demands. The concept was that the human was not designed to do close work, the implication being that the eyes were distal receptors and for the purpose of seeing at a distance, not at near. It was further implied that as man developed and began to deal with symbols, eventually referred to as reading and writing, the unnaturalness of this type of task resulted in impairment. This was a neat way of rationalizing the emerging of visual disabilities, but the rationale is not consistent with physiology and behavior.

There is no such thing as a nearpoint visual problem. Problems are not created because of near work activities. The problem is not in the task. There is no problem in the eyes. It is more appropriate and consistent to state that near-centered demands may be the stressor-agent producing a persistent stress requiring adaptation. This adaptation is adverse in that bodily structure alteration is required to permit maintenance of function with the least expenditure of energy.

The non-embedded syndrome of the stress-induced visual problem, including the shift toward increased esophoria, is an example of visual performance with increased effort and energy expenditure. In contrast, the embedded syndrome, with shift from esophoria to increased exophoria, is representative of habituated performance with less effort and energy expenditure.

"Myopia may be viewed as the adaptation of fight, and reduced visual efficiency as flight."

At this point, our first two questions of what is stress and what is THE stress have been addressed. But, where is the stress? It is not in the task. It is not in the eyes. As Selye said, it is in the body, but being even more specific, stress induced in the visual process is initially demonstrated in orientation processes, with increased energy demanded to sustain balance with gravity and the task. This results in increased tonicity of musculature required for sustaining postural balancing mechanisms. With the persistency of the stress, the body must adapt to reduce this stress, i.e., grow along a line of stress to reduce stress. The hyper-tonicity must be reduced in order to permit function with minimum effort. This is the resulting adverse adaptation and viewed optometrically within the syndrome of the stress-induced visual problem as either the primary adaptation of myopia or the adaptation of reduced visual efficiency. Walter B. Cannon described adaptation as either fight or flight.[6] Myopia may be viewed as the adaptation of fight and reduced visual efficiency as flight.

In reality, all visual dysfunction, whether the result of interference in development or interference in that which has been developed, may be viewed as stress-induced. It is simply for convenience and categorization (and possibly for lack of a better label) that we refer to one as the vision development problem due to thwarting of development, and the other the stress-induced visual problem. There is no question as to difference in behavior and performance as viewed optometrically between these two categories, and the clinical approaches will vary with etiology. But in the last analysis, the thwarting of development is also a stressor-agent, and the result is an adaptation to a persisting stress.

The goal of life is not freedom from stress since, as Selye has so well demonstrated, stress is essential to life. The goal of life, on the other hand, could well be freedom from effort and persistent-stressor agents. From an ideal viewpoint, this is the goal of the behavioral approach for patients. This is preventive vision care. This is provided as a product of programming vision care. The fundamental role of the counter-stress lenses, whether for prevention or protection, control and maintenance, is to reduce persistent stress. This in turn permits the person to function with minimal effort required for orientation so that maximum energy is available for the purposes of deriving meaning and directing action.

References
1. Weiner H. Communicating for Success. Curriculum II. Santa Ana, CA: Optometric Extension Program, 1981-1982.
2. Selye H. Stress without Distress. New York: J. P. Lippincott Co., 1974.

3. Selye H. The Stress of Life. New York: McGraw-Hill Book Co., Inc., 1956.
4. Selye H. The Story of the Adaptation Syndrome. Montreal: Acta, Inc., Med. Publ., 1952.
5. Harmon DB. Notes on a Dynamic Theory of Vision. Published by the author, 1958.
6. Cannon WB. The Wisdom of the Body. New York: W. W. Norton & Co., Inc., 1932.

Recommended Reading
1. Kraskin RA. Vision Training in Action. Santa Ana, CA: Optometric Extension Program, Series 1, 2, 3, 1965-68.
2. Barstow R, Kraskin RA. Practice Management. Santa Ana, CA: Optometric Extension Program, Series 28, 1960-61.

APPENDIX A
Optometric Evaluation, Comments and Recommendations for Mr. CLH, age at exam time 22-6

October 13

1. Stress Induced Visual Problem B2, partially embedded: reduced visual efficiency
2. The examination for ocular pathology and abnormality was negative
3. No prior vision care
4. Sees clearly at far and near
5. No focus lag reported
6. No visual discomfort reported
7. Has allergy problems, which seem to affect eyes
8. Claims to be fast reader but is aware of need to "reread" for comprehension
9. Some difficulty with concentration
10. College student, 2nd year—communications major
11. Works with film and movies
12. Has been aware of some difficulty in focusing with camera recently
13. Unaided visual acuity at far: R 20/25, L slow 20/25 to 20/20, OU 20/20; at near: R & L both 20/20
14. Ocular motility: poor
15. Telebinocular DB series: suppressions, 3 balls unstable and eso at far and near
16. No ocular defects: normal hyperopia
17. Imbalance in near vision function
18. Responds to plus on stresspoint retinoscope.
19. The optometric evaluation of the collected data and information reveals the partially embedded syndrome of the stress-induced visual problem associated with reduced visual efficiency, resulting in limitations and restriction in information processing. More recent increased demands have created increased awareness of limitations and resulting manifestations of awareness of some symptoms, which were not manifest in the past. The dysfunction has existed since earlier school days.

Optometric Care Program Alternatives

1. Conventional: 20/20, healthy eyes, no ocular defects; do nothing
2. Functional: control and minimal improvement: provide appropriate counter-stress lenses in dual focus form to be used for all visually near-centered activities. The use of such lenses will reduce current stress, permitting more effective use of present abilities, increased sustaining ability and minimal gains in efficiency. Expect improvement in ease of functioning, and increased ability to meet demands of camera

focusing. Return for reevaluation examination in three months. $310.00 (Note: this fee reflects the author's fees in the early 1980's when this was first published.)

Visual training: To develop and restore the desirable and adequate visual abilities, and the freedom to utilize these abilities as a product of developing a more effective and efficient visual system. Anticipate improvement in all visually oriented activities such as reading efficiency, etc. Predict 6-8 months.

CHAPTER 11
Compensatory Lenses and Postural Alterations

Recognition of the visual process as the dominant process of human behavior is fundamental to the behavioral concept of vision.

The constructive alteration and control of behavior by the optometric utilization of lenses has been the underlying theme of this book. It is important to appreciate that the imposition of any lens before an eye will alter behavior, constructively or otherwise. The goal of the behavioral approach is to use lenses, if at all possible, for constructive purposes. The last chapter on patient management in the context of behavioral approach to optometric care demonstrated that the final decision and selection of the level of vision care rests with the patient (not the optometrist) as a product of offering every patient alternatives of optometric care.

The constructive use of lenses can be described as the application and utilization of lenses to enhance visual performance and protect the integrity of visual performance. Obviously, such lenses will not contribute deliberately to the degradation of visual behavior; this would be counterproductive and possibly destructive. The fundamental notion of the constructive use of lenses is peculiar to the behavioral concept of vision.

Previous chapters have addressed the constructive use of lenses, primarily counter-stress lenses (usually low plus lenses), and yoked prisms for the following purposes:

1. Prevention (counter-stress lenses)
2. Protection, control and maintenance (counter-stress lenses)
3. Enhancement (counter-stress lenses and/or yoked prisms)

The use of such lenses constructively alters behavior.

Alteration of visual behavior is not limited to the utilization of stress-relieving plus lenses and yoked prisms.

In the first chapter of this book the author listed the seven fundamental tenets of the dynamic concept of vision. Tenet #6 suggested that the purposes of lens use were prevention, protection, remediation, compensation and enhancement. Given that remediation and enhancement are identical, the use of lenses for everything except compensation has been previously considered in these chapters. While the consideration of compensatory lenses is not related to the major purpose of this book, it cannot be ignored because compensatory lenses also alter behavior, either constructively or otherwise.

"All ocular defects are reflections of postural alterations."

Compensatory lenses were defined in the first chapter as lenses, which compensate for existing identifiable and measurable "refractive" conditions. The only justification from the behavioral concept viewpoint to prescribe compensatory lenses is if utilization of such lenses is constructive to behavior and performance. When professional judgment recognizes this constructive value, the guideline to be followed is that the prescription must always equal the minimal degree of compensation required to provide constructive benefit. Inappropriate utilization of such lenses can be counterproductive and can cause additional adverse behavior and maladaptation.

Examples of compensatory lenses are (1) concave lenses to compensate for myopia, (2) convex lenses to compensate for adverse hyperopia, (3) cylindrical lenses to compensate for astigmatism, (4) differences in lenses to compensate for anisometropia and antimetropia, and (5) vertical prisms to compensate for vertical deviances.

Also, this author has suggested that all ocular defects are reflections of postural alterations. The above-listed conditions for which compensatory lenses can be prescribed are examples of various alterations in body posture reflected optometrically as ocular defects.

The stress of life was discussed in the previous chapter. It was noted that stress is essential for life; stress was defined as the nonspecific response of the body to a demand placed upon it. Contrary to popular usage of the word, stress is not necessarily negative or undesirable. Stress is a necessity for constructive performance from the positive point of view. In other words, stress demands performance; behavior is triggered by stress. Transient stress is constructive and positive, and the living organism is designed to meet transient stress with constructive changes in behavior. However, persistent stress is negative; the result is adverse adaptation—maladaptation—yet essential for survival. In his later years, Selye differentiated between positive and negative stress by coining the term eustress to designate the positive; he used the term distress to define the negative non-constructive change in function—the maladaptation resultant.

Like stress, compensatory lenses are also endowed with a negative connotation. Again there are both positive and negative sides to the issue. Compensatory lenses are significant if their utilization results in constructive performance, thus enhancing behavior. The implication is that such utilization does not result in an additional adverse adaptation, but provides benefits significant to the person's whole being.

On the other hand, use of compensatory lenses is negative if such use does not result in constructive performance or if such use results in additional maladaptation. When compensatory lenses are prescribed and do not provide constructive change, adverse adaptation frequently results. Additionally, inappropriate use of compensatory lenses results in adverse adaptation. Compensatory lenses become a stressor agent and induce a persistent stress when used under conditions different from those in which such lenses can be significant or when not significant to the performance of a person. This will result in adverse adaptation and further maladaptation. Generally, the arbitrary prescribing of compensatory lenses will result in undesirable and non-constructive changes in behavior.

An optometric finding or combination of findings such as myopia, hyperopia, astigmatism, anisometropia or hyperphoria does not suggest automatically that compensation for such conditions is required or constructive. Much more must be appreciated relative to the needs of the person and the benefits desired. Chapter 7 explored myopia from the behavioral viewpoint. Recall that myopia varies with the viewing distance. If myopia is revealed in the #7 (subjective) finding, it is significantly less or none at all at near. Assuming that there is benefit to be gained by the patient's use of minus lenses beyond near space, the use of such lenses for near-centered demands induces stress in the body and requires an adverse adaptation—identified as increased myopia.

It is not unusual to prescribe lenses for constant wear equivalent to the #7 (subjective) finding from the conventional point of view. The rationale is that this finding represents a "refractive error." If unaided visual acuity is standard 20/20 and the #7 (subjective) is in plus, the arbitrary prescribing of equivalent lenses for constant wear can result in a reduction of unaided visual acuity and a need for periodic increases in the plus to maintain standard acuity. This is not in the interest of constructive change in performance; in fact, quite the contrary. Adverse hyperopia results from stress triggered by the utilization of such lenses acting as a stressor agent.

Another example of induced adverse hyperopia is the result of the patient's misuses of single vision reading lenses. Frequently, the patient is provided with appropriate counter-stress lenses for near-centered demands but in single vision form. This is not unusual at all from the conventional point of view. It is the procedure followed with early presbyopes. Single vision lenses are very difficult to use and to avoid misuse. In this case, misuse is described as the periodic unintentional viewing at far through the lenses. For example, the patient looks upward from close work when attention is called across the room; the patient then removes the glasses because what he sees is blurred and annoying. Such misuse is stress inducing and it can result in demand for adverse adaptation with a manifestation of adverse hyperopia. This is self-manufactured hyperopia and certainly it is not in the best interest of the patient or the patient's performance and behavior. From the positive point of view, when such lenses are required for near-centered demands and the patient reveals this proneness, Plano add bifocals or half-eye lenses are necessary to ensure constructive benefits and to avoid adverse unintentional adaptation.

Similar consideration must be given also to the prescribing of cylindrical lenses, differences in lenses for either eye, and vertical prism. Insight into astigmatism, anisometropia, and vertical deviances will reveal appropriate guidelines to prescribe and when not to prescribe from the behavioral concept viewpoint. The mere fact that astigmatism, anisometropia, and/or hyperphoria exist does not justify prescription of such lenses. Such compensation can be significant to constructive performance and, if so, should be prescribed.

However, such compensation should be avoided if the use of such lenses contributes to additional maladaptation. It has not been unusual, for example, to prescribe vertical prism when hyperphoria is revealed. After a period of use, the vertical phoria is greater and more prism is prescribed. The question should be asked whether or not this has been constructive or whether this is any different than progressive myopia? The optometrist advocating a behavioral approach answers "NO" to both questions.

Assuming professional judgment recognizes constructive value, the basic guideline for the optometrist prescribing compensatory lenses from a behavioral approach is that such prescription equals the minimal degree of compensation required for performance and patient benefit, and that such lens utilization is controlled to prevent misuse.

Near-centered demands and the thwarting of vision development have been demonstrated to be the prime stressor agents resulting in disability in the visual process. But, manifestation of dysfunction in the visual system is not limited to stress induced by the previously mentioned stressor agents.

Anything creating a persistent alteration in body balancing mechanics and musculature associated with posture can lead to asymmetric maladaptations of the body, which are revealed as postural warps. Such stressor agents and resulting asymmetries can be reflected overtly in the visual process and identified in the course of the routine optometric examination. The stress induced by the persistence of near-centered demands has been discussed in the preceding chapter

Perhaps the most common stressor agents associated with the maladaptation and reflected as astigmatism, anisometropia, and vertical phoria are environmental forces such as lighting and postural influences related to chair and desk heights in visually demanding school and occupational activities. Postural warps related to congenital defects, as well as restraints and restrictions in movement-coordination development in the early years of child development, can be reflected in the visual process. Traumatic conditions affecting posturing musculature often will be reflected in the course of the optometric examination. As an example, it is not unusual for a vertical imbalance to be revealed following an automobile accident that results in whiplash. This vertical imbalance can result in temporary vertical diplopia.

Additional analysis will reveal that any stressor agent inducing stress which results in alteration of the alignment of the head, such as head turn, head tilt, or a combination of head tilt and head turn, can be reflected optometrically as astigmatism, anisometropia, vertical phoria or combinations of these adaptations. These are examples of the often quoted Harmon statement that an organism grows along the line of stress so as to reduce stress, the process of adaptation, and in these cases, maladaptation.

Alteration of head alignment can be the result of external influences, such as lighting in a working environment, which affects the posturing of the head. Inappropriate distribution of lighting can force a person to alter position in an attempt to balance the light distribution and create, in turn, the asymmetric positioning of the head. This can result in one eye closer to the task than the other or one eye higher than the other in relation to the task. This leads to asymmetry of activity of the neck musculature (the sternomastoid) which feeds downward, affecting the musculature of the upper back and the posturing musculature of the lower back, resulting in rotation and tilt of the pelvis. Recall from the discussion involving lateral yoked prisms that rotation of the eyes is antagonistic to rotation of the pelvis. For example, when eyes rotate left, pelvis rotates right. Another way of stating the same thing is that the pelvis rotates in the direction of the head or vice versa. The resulting manifestation of identified ocular defect is dependent on how the total posturing musculature is affected and adapts.

This process is the same in reverse. The stressor agent imposes itself initially in the basic posturing center associated with the lower back and pelvis. The influence and process of alteration, change and adaptation are the same if the stressor agent imposes itself at any level other than head and pelvis, such as in upper back or neck. As examples, the physical influence of seating arrangements in a working environment can result in a rotated pelvis, which ultimately feeds upward and results in a misalignment of the head. The same is true of congenital defects and developmental impediments affecting posturing mechanisms and movement coordination development. Likewise, trauma, such as whiplash affecting upper back and neck, would induce the same process of change. It is important to emphasize that all ocular defects are reflections of alterations in posture. However, not all alterations in posture are reflected as ocular defects. The optometric evidence of an identifiable ocular "defect" denotes that there is a postural equivalent related to the ocular defect; yet the absence of identifiable ocular defects should not presume the absence of postural alterations. It can be assumed such alteration will be revealed in the optometric examination the longer the postural alteration exists and the more adaptation takes place.

It is appropriate at this point to recall the words of the late A. M. Skeffington, O.D. "It takes time," he said, "for protoplasm to show trace." Some readers may recall the amazing demonstrations by D. B. Harmon, Ph.D., who, by postural analysis, could state within a reasonable degree of accuracy (and more often alarmingly accurate) the refractive status of any given person.

Astigmatism, a postural alteration

In response to a patient's question, "What is ... ?", optometrists almost unanimously agree that the term astigmatism is the most difficult clinical term to define or to describe (and be comfortable with the answer). From an optical point of view, if nothing else, optometrists have within themselves an insight, but it is extremely difficult to define or describe to a layman. Historically, the word astigmatism was "sold" to the public and became generic as a condition. In response to the question, "What is wrong with my eyes?", the patient was answered with the term astigmatism. And it was accepted much like other labels are accepted—as conditions in the health field— although the public may not have or have even sought a definition of the condition.

The term is so common that it is used frequently by the layman but still mispronounced. How often will a patient exclaim? "I was told I had stigmatism." It has always been interesting to this author that no other clinical terms, such as myopia and hyperopia, are part of the vocabulary of the average person. Rather, the average person knows and uses terminology such as nearsightedness and farsightedness. Perhaps astigmatism conveys the notion of some mysterious condition. Although not mysterious, approaches to vision care other than the behavioral point of view consider astigmatism as a condition—a defect.

The behavioral approach views the existence of astigmatism (as well as other ocular defects) as representative of change or alteration of posture rather than conditions in themselves. The optometric evidence of an ocular defect represents the individual's adaptation required to maintain the integrity of performance as one grows along a line of stress to reduce stress. Recall Tenet #1, "The visual process is dominant." Inherent in this understanding is the recognition and appreciation that 20% of the optic nerve fibers, representing as much as 85% of the retinal nerve cells, pass through the superior colliculus and go to the posturing mechanisms of the body. Posturing and balancing mechanisms are part and parcel of the visual process.

The following statements further emphasize this significance:

1. "The visual world and the gravitational world are inseparable components of a unified perceptual world," according to James G. Taylor, in his book, *The Behavioral Basis of Perception*, Yale University Press, 1962.
2. "The body is always the locus of perception and...the quality of an individual's perception depends directly on how his body is functioning," according to Michael Gelb, in his book, *Body Learning*, Delilah Books, 1981.

Historically, astigmatism has been classified as "with" the rule, "against" the rule and oblique. Apparently such classification emerged initially as a product of clinical evidence in that astigmia with minus axis at 180 was more commonly evidenced and, thus, earned the label—"with" the rule. Minus cylinder axis 90 was more unusual; therefore, it was "against" the rule. Anything other than cylinder minus axis 180 or 90 was oblique.

Today most clinicians would wonder if the labels should have been reversed since it would seem that more "against" the rule astigmatism exists than "with" the rule. These latter observations have been made for 30 or 40 years. What could have changed in ourselves or in our environment to result in an increased evidence of "against" the rule astigmatism? Additionally, it has been revealed clinically that "against" the rule astigmatism usually affects visual acuity more than "with" the rule. It is not unusual that "against" the rule astigmatism is evident in the early stage of myopia adaptation—perhaps as a forerunner to the manifestation of myopia. This is not the case for "with" the rule astigmatism.

Optometrists engaged in visual training often observe another interesting detail. That is, as the visual training program progresses, the initially revealed astigmatism is the most rapid manifestation to be altered in the realm of refractive status.

Evidence suggests that any identified astigmatism is an ocular manifestation of asymmetric muscular involvement in posturing mechanisms; it may evolve as the result of inadequacy in development, environmental forces and even trauma. Regardless of the stressor agent, the locus of involvement in the posturing musculature reflects and creates the nature of the astigmatism.

It is critical at this time to restate a paragraph from earlier in the text:

> *"Information processing is experienced as movements—both overt and covert. These movement patterns are described as orientation and localization. Orientation describes the resultant of the body's coming to balance with gravity and with the task. This involves the posturing mechanisms associated with these activities. On the other hand, localization is a derivative of the body's coming to balance on the task and manipulating the task. It should be noted that the commitment of coming to balance with the task demand is common both to orientation and localization. In terms of balancing mechanisms, orientation involves the lower back muscles; localization involves the upper back and neck musculature."*

Without going into musculature detail, kinesiology, and specific components of posturing mechanisms, it appears that the locus of "against" the rule astigmatism is within the movement pattern of orientation—the lower back musculature. Likewise, "with" the rule astigmatism reflects an alteration in localization and it involves the upper back. It is highly likely that any manifestation of oblique astigmatism is evidence of interference in the posturing musculature of orientation and localization. It is also likely that the optometric measurement revealed is a vector resultant of the forces involved in the musculature and mechanism of posture creating such torques.

"Astigmatism must never be viewed or interpreted as a condition in itself. Any evidence of astigmatism would be a reflection of an alteration in body posture."

If this is true, there must be mechanisms involved, which permit the feed-forward of motor signals that result in an alteration of the optics of the eye, especially the cornea and the crystalline lens. It has been well known for years that the cornea is not a static structure and that it is quite plastic. Evidence now reveals, for example, that the extraocular muscles can respond in their pairing and action in such a way as to create torque on the cornea. This action can be the reason for manifestation of "with" the rule astigmatism beginning with the adverse activity of the upper back. Of course, the foregoing is speculation at this time —speculation that corresponds to fact to some degree—as well as notion.

The clinical manifestation of astigmatism must never be viewed or interpreted as a condition in itself, as a visual problem, or as the cause of a visual problem. Such manifestation might or might not reflect a disability in the visual process. On the other hand, if the above speculation were true, any evidence of astigmatism would be a reflection of an alteration in body posture which, in itself, could be transient and not evidence a disability.

As an example, the studies involving the investigation of child and vision development indicate that a child could reveal transient astigmatism at certain ages and stages of development—at one age, "with" the rule, and at another age, "against" the rule. Yet, this is not evidence of a vision dysfunction or a postural problem. On the other hand, these observations of transient astigmatism, as well as numerous other transient ocular revelations noted in watching vision and child development, are nothing more than the ocular manifestation of changes and periods of growth and development within the motor system of the total child.

Another example of transience was revealed dramatically some years ago by a study at The Illinois College of Optometry under the direction of Leo Manas, O.D. A group of optometric students were examined optometrically prior to taking final examinations, and then immediately at the conclusion of the final examinations, and then again some time later. The study revealed that there was an obvious high degree of manifestation of "against" the rule astigmatism immediately following final examinations, which had not existed prior to the final examinations. This astigmatism was not revealed when this same group was examined some weeks following the final examinations.

The important point to be gained from this discussion is that evidence of astigmatism alone does not mean that the suspected astigmatism is a condition. More importantly, it should not be concluded automatically that it is a representation of a condition requiring intervention. Much more about the total behavior must be known other than mere indications of an astigmatism. In other words, the mere evidence of astigmatism is not license to prescribe compensatory lenses, let alone evidence of the need for any form of optometric program of care.

The commonly accepted and standard optometric means to determine the presence of astigmatism is through retinoscopy observation and the subjective (#7) probe of the analytical examination. The identification of meridional difference revealed in any one or more of the various retinoscopy procedures is clinically significant to understand the visual process and the performance of a given patient. In no way is it indicative that cylindrical lenses should be provided. Simply, it is indicative that astigmatism is revealed for whatever reason under the conditions of the particular procedure. The behavioral optometrist is aware of the possibility of the high variability in meridional difference that can be revealed between the numerous retinoscopy procedures employed in the course of the diagnostic examination. An optometrist following a behavioral approach to optometric care also knows that no retinoscopic finding itself is a prescribable lens formula for compensatory purposes.

Likewise, the variance in astigmatic findings that might exist between retinoscopy observations and the subjective is well known. Because a given degree of astigmatism is observed with the farpoint retinoscopic procedure, for example, it does not follow that the same degree and axis will be revealed in the #7 (subjective) finding. Also, the retinoscopy finding is frequently spherical, but the subjective probe results in an identifiable degree of astigmatism.

From the behavioral point of view, the optometrist gives consideration to a prescription of cylindrical lenses only if astigmatism is revealed in the subjective probe (#7), and then, only if the use of such lenses is constructive to the patient's performance and needs. The revelation of astigmatism itself does not justify such prescribing.

The subjective probe is critical. The procedure itself, the means to determine astigmatism, and its inclusion as part of the final subjective finding are critical. The results of this probe can vary depending upon the clinician's procedure for doing the #7 (subjective). This author insists that any cylinder incorporated as an element in the final finding is earned by the patient. The following represents the standardized subjective probe of this author in the course of the optometric examination for astigmatism:

Following the #5 (retinoscopy at 20 inches), the patient's left eye is occluded. Cylinder, if seen on #5, is removed and the patient views a blurred 20/50 horizontal row of letters through the gross spherical element of the #5 finding. The plus lens power is reduced in quarter diopter steps until the 20/50 letters are identifiable. The same is then repeated for the left eye while viewing a different row of 20/50 letters. The astigmatic sunburst dial is presented to the patient while viewing with the left eye. Meridional differences, if any, are noted to determine power and axis meridian. The rotary T target is exposed in the appropriate position if difference exists and cylinder is added until the T is equalized. The same is repeated with the right eye viewing. Proceed immediately to the right eye if no difference exists initially when viewing the sunburst dial.

When completing the probes with astigmatic dials, a horizontal row of 20/50 letters is exposed to the right eye and the plus is reduced in quarter diopter steps until the letters are identified. If cylinder is in the phoropter, the standard Jackson crossed cylinder test for both axis and power refinement is done. If cylinder still remains, the final determinant is purely subjective in that the cylinder is reduced in quarter diopter steps to note if the patient is aware of a difference in the clarity of the letters. The final power of the cylinder is that level which, if reduced one quarter diopter more, affects the clarity of the 20/25 letters. The same is repeated for the left eye. The acuity quality between the two eyes is balanced and equalized at the 20/25 level. Then, a 20/20 horizontal row of letters is exposed under binocular conditions and the plus is reduced binocularly in quarter diopter steps until the letters are seen clearly. The final #7 (subjective) is represented by the combination of lenses (sphere and cylinder) remaining in the phoropter at this time. If cylinder remains, this is considered the astigmatic degree that is significant but not necessarily to be prescribed or provided in a lens formula for the patient.

The question—when to prescribe or when not to prescribe cylinder compensating for astigmatism—remains. Hopefully, the following will provide the reader with the insight and answers to this question.

The sole purpose of prescribing any compensatory lens combination is to provide the patient with a more effective input to instigate the process of vision. The ultimate change in the optical mechanism of the eye (viewed as an ocular defect) exists as a product of the adverse alteration of body posture—the resultant being an inappropriate or inadequate distribution of light and, subsequently, a decrement in the quality of the signals triggered by the light distribution. Thus, the information inherent in the signals is denigrated because of the increased noise. The compensatory lens restores the more desirable and adequate light distribution, and thus, in turn, the noise level is reduced and the quality of the signal for information is enhanced.

Recall our definition of vision—the deriving of meaning and directing of action as a product of processing information triggered by a selected band of radiant energy. The degraded information can result in a lessened ability to derive meaning and direct action easily and effectively with such manifestation as a limitation in visual acuity, restriction in utilization of the binocular input, and general inefficiency. When this is the case, compensatory lenses could be prescribed, especially if the process is not alterable by other more positive means.

In considering the necessity for prescribing compensatory cylindrical lenses, the behavioral approach directs the optometrist to appreciate the status of adaptation and the degree of embeddedness. The less embedded the visual behavioral pattern, the less reason to consider astigmatic compensation, if a positive behavioral approach is taken with the application of stress-relieving lenses.

"Unless required for visual acuity, any use of cylindrical lenses would be delimiting."

There would be no justification to incorporate compensatory lenses in the final prescription if the goal is protection, control, maintenance, and/or enhancement. Unless required for visual acuity, any use of cylindrical lenses would be delimiting. On the other hand, the more embedded the status, the more it might be necessary to incorporate compensatory cylinder in any prescription. Of course, this depends upon the significance of such lenses on patient performance and need. The experienced clinician is aware of the greater significance to performance when the behavior is embedded and reveals "against" the rule cylinder as compared to "with" the rule cylinder.

Case Example

Tom O represents an excellent illustration. He was 17 years old when he was initially examined. An excellent student, he had become aware of some difficulty seeing the chalkboards. Without listing the data of the complete analytical examination and related performance tests, the evaluation of the data revealed a non-embedded pattern.

Unaided visual acuity was: OD 20/25, OS 20/25, OU 20/25. The subjective (#7) was: OD -0.75 x 90, 20/20; OS -1.00 x 70, 20/20. The #1 alternative, the conventional approach, would have called for prescribing compensatory lenses equivalent to the #7 for constant wear. The #2 alternative, the functional approach, was, likewise, the recommendation for lenses to be worn constantly (but a prescription quite different from that of alternative #1) on a temporary basis rather than a permanent one as provided in alternative #1. Assuming proper patient cooperation, the predictable benefits were excellent at this stage of non-embeddedness. The #3 alternative, of course, was visual training. The patient selected the #2 alternative: the prescription of OU Plano with 4 bases-up yoked prisms, add +1.00.

Tom returned for his programmed progress case study three months later. He was no longer aware of any limitation in visual acuity. Unaided visual acuity was 20/20 right eye, left eye and both eyes. The subjective (#7) was OU Plano. Absolutely no astigmatism was revealed. It was obvious that Tom was in an early stage of myopic adaptation when seen initially. The process was reversed with the use of the stress-relieving lenses. The lenses were not altered, and he was asked to continue the use of the lenses for all indoor activity, rather than constantly. He will continue this until he reveals plus in the subjective (#7), at which time the prism will be removed and the appropriate plus in dual focus form will be used for near work for preventive purposes only.

Anisometropia and vertical imbalance

In the first chapter of this book it was noted that the late A. M. Skeffington, O.D., former Director of Education for the Optometric Extension Program Foundation, had a unique ability to raise the most thought-provoking questions of his colleagues and associates. "What is the value of binocularity?" was one such question.

From the point of view inherent in conventional wisdom, the answer to this question was fairly standardized. Primarily, it related to (1) stereopsis, (2) assumptions related to the notion of binocular problems and (3) the implied concept that one sees with an eye or a pair of eyes. However, such a standardized (and accepted) answer was inconsistent both with reality and emerging factual information. Such an answer was inadequate; nor did it satisfy the then emerging dynamic functional concept of vision. Thus, the question was raised.

Conventional concepts implied that so-called depth perception was a product primarily of man's ability to see with two eyes—the implication being that stereopsis was normal seeing. In addition, standardized texts assumed that additional cues derived from either eye alone contributed to the totality and quality of depth perception. Such cues, referred to as monocular cues, were the rationale to explain depth perception when either one eye was occluded or in the one-eyed person. Nevertheless, the terms stereopsis and depth perception were used interchangeably. For example, the index of Zoethout's text, Physiological Optics, refers to stereopsis when you look up depth perception.

The accommodative-convergence physiologic optic concept of vision provided such labels as convergence and divergence problems from which was derived the general notion of binocular problems. The implication is that one has a so-called binocular problem because one has two eyes not working together. This further implies that one is subject to dysfunction because they have two eyes. (If this were true, perhaps the human being would have been better off if he had only one eye.) The use of the term binocular problems suggests that a monocular problem might be also a converse disability. Interestingly, however, a current search of some optometric college curriculums has revealed that courses bear the title, "binocular dysfunction" or "binocular problems." Nowhere has this author found a course labeled "monocular dysfunction."

The suggestion that one sees with one or two eyes, e.g., that vision is in the eye(s), is common to all conventional wisdom concepts. Although still limiting (as related to the behavioral concept), Gordon Walls's statement that vision is a product of a simple eye and a complex brain was a giant step forward.

Admittedly, the conventional concepts recognize that brain contributes to vision, but such concepts still suggest that there are two components—the eyes and the brain. Thus, the terms monocularity and binocularity were created. These suggest that monocular vision is seeing with one eye and binocular vision is seeing with two eyes. (It is implied that these terms are conditions of output.)

As an aside (yet significant to this discussion) is the fact that the notion of monocular vision training and binocular visual training was derived in the earlier developing years of visual training. This also led to the notion of monocular and binocular visual skills as if skill was in an eye or in a pair of eyes. In fact, a new (temporary) term was coined for descriptive purposes, which was *biocular*, because there were visual training procedures that were not monocular or binocular but incorporated procedures under conditions of prism dissociation. Thus, in those days, we had monocular, biocular, and binocular training procedures and viewed them as a hierarchy of a visual training program—implying the development of monocular, biocular, and binocular visual skills—skills of eyes—again suggesting that these terms related to conditions of output.

"We do not see with an eye or a pair of eyes."

Dr. Skeffington's question on the value of binocularity arose as the inadequacy, inconsistency and incompatibility of the foregoing implications began to emerge. It climaxed with the recognition that the terms "monocularity" and "binocularity" were perfectly acceptable and usable terms but not as adjectives related to vision, seeing or output. With the emerging appreciation that vision is output, vision is motor, and that vision, itself, is an emergent (the deriving of meaning and directing of action), it became obvious that we could not speak of "monocular vision" or "binocular vision," let alone "biocular vision." This recognized that we do not see with an eye or a pair of eyes.

The eyes are designed to accept and distribute light over the retina. The retina, acting as a transducer, triggers an input to activate the process of vision. The terms monocular and binocular were perfectly appropriate to describe the conditions of input. Monocularity describes the activation of the visual process triggered by an input derived from light being admitted to one eye. Binocularity, likewise, describes the activation of the visual process triggered by inputs derived from light being admitted to both eyes, dissociated or otherwise. Appreciating this led to the fact that there was no longer a need to persist with the term biocular in the behavioral concept vocabulary. It is absolutely meaningless. So what is the value of binocularity? These chapters have continuously emphasized that the fundamental characteristic of the behavioral concept is the recognition and appreciation of the role of the 20% of optic nerve fibers that lead to the posturing mechanisms of the body.

Further, it should be appreciated that the only animals that have eyes in the front of the head are those capable of standing on their hind legs. However, this does not imply that two eyes are a necessity in order to stand on one's hind legs. On the other hand, as will soon be evident, the mechanism involved to stand on hind legs will be altered and different if one had only one eye. The activation of the visual process depends on light-related input from which is derived orientation and localization. The musculature involved in orientation and localization, therefore, depends on the input, especially the input related to the all-important 20% of nerve fibers leading to the superior colliculus and to the posturing mechanisms of the body which permit coming to balance with gravity and the task.

"The primary value of binocularity relates to balancing mechanisms associated with orientation."

It would appear that the primary value of binocularity relates to balancing mechanisms of the bilateral system associated with orientation. In addition to establishing balance with the task (which is common to both orientation and localization), manipulation of the task is a function of localization. This is a higher order function and it is the processing of information triggered primarily by signals related to the more commonly considered 80% of optic nerve fibers, which pass through the lateral geniculates.

Here lies the second value of binocularity in that redundancy, a recognized need of any information processing system, is provided to permit the most effective and efficient means to derive meaning and direct action. The two inputs triggered by the two eyes, each conveying similar information, provide this benefit of redundancy. This is but one example of redundancy in the total process but is undoubtedly a most significant one. Another would be the feed-forward information arising as the product of coming to balance with gravity and the task, which contributes to the manipulation of the task.

In summation, therefore, it appears that the value of binocularity relates to maintaining the integrity of a bilateral system and the insurance of redundancy—both of which are essential for efficient and effective vision—the deriving of meaning and directing of action.

"The second value of binocularity...redundancy...to derive meaning and direct action."

Binocularity is the provision of input triggered by light-related energy to both eyes. How the system utilizes this input is another matter. It depends primarily on the adequacy of orientation. Within recent years, Colwyn Trevarthen, a psycho-biologist at the University of Edinburgh, has concluded (using different language) that there are two modes of seeing. One is information to orient in space at large, and the second is to explore local structure for identity determination. The former he calls "ambient vision" and the latter, "focal vision." Analysis of his work reveals that when he speaks of ambient vision, he refers to that which we have labeled orientation; focal vision is localization. His reference to seeing actually refers to inputs related to the two aspects of the leads emanating from the optic nerves, one leading to lower centers and the other to the higher center. The adequacy and effectiveness of one depends directly on the adequacy of the other.

Appreciation of the foregoing is essential to understand further and to accept that which is inherent in the behavioral concept as well as to understand the guidelines related to the use of lenses within this concept—no matter what the condition. This is particularly significant when consideration is given to additional alterations in posture reflected optometrically as anisometropia and vertical imbalance. For the present, we shall consider anisometropia.

Optometrically, we shall define anisometropia as a condition in which the refractive status differs between the two eyes—that is, one eye is more hyperopic than the other or one eye is more myopic than the other. The term antimetropia is customarily used to differentiate the condition in which one eye is myopic and the other hyperopic, but this is just a special term, of course, and in reality this situation is another example of anisometropia in general, and it will be considered as such. The asymmetrical refractive status is a reflection of an asymmetric postural status of the body. It represents a rotation about the gravitational axis of the body, and more specifically, a rotation of the pelvis. A lateral rotation of the pelvis is accompanied by some degree of pelvic tilt—a secondary shoulder alteration, usually with the shoulder lowering on the side of the raised pelvis. In addition, there exists a head turn in the direction of the eye revealing the greater ocular "defect." Such postural asymmetry may be induced or created by a thwarting of development, which would be a manifestation of a vision development problem. More commonly, however, such postural asymmetries are the result of environmental forces over time, such as lighting and seating arrangements. These create body torques associated with the socially compulsive biologically unacceptable visually near-centered demands, particularly those involving handwriting activities.

Recognizing the significance of these environmental influencing factors, the optometrist providing a behavioral approach to optometric care, who by definition is concerned with prevention, strives to provide visual hygiene guidance. Such materials as OEP's Visual Hygiene Pamphlet and the Journal of the American Optometric Association reprint, "Easier and More Productive Study and Desk Work," by A. W. Francke, O.D., and W. J. Kaplan, O.D. (both available from OEP) are essential, supportive information for all patients.

If the condition exists, the behavioral approach to the patient's optometric care depends on the status of the condition in relationship to the desires of the patient.

The diagnostic examination will reveal the condition and the total status of the condition. The evaluation of the examination data will reveal the status of the patient's visual behavior from which directives of appropriate optometric care will be derived and benefits anticipated. Obviously, the examination data will reveal if the condition of anisometropia exists and to what degree. The data will reveal how effectively the patient utilizes the binocular inputs. The data also will reveal if the utilization of the binocular input can be improved either by altering the patient behavior or by altering the quality of the binocular input. The quality of the binocular input would be altered by utilization of compensatory lenses—that is, lenses that compensate for the anisometropia to whatever degree required.

Altering patient behavior would be induced primarily by lenses, such as stress-relieving plus and/or yoked prisms. The significance or lack of significance of either compensatory lenses or therapeutic lenses would be determined by visual performance observations. This would indicate the effect of such lenses on binocular demand activities, such as Polaroid tests (Wirt, Titmus, etc.), Telebinocular stereo tests, analytical examination probes, such as phorias and ductions, and the Harmon Square test. Stresspoint retinoscopy will reveal the availability or lack of an indicated counter-stress lens formula. Undoubtedly, there are numerous other means to investigate the significance of lenses other than those, which this author utilizes in the course of a routine diagnostic examination.

Assuming patient desire, the behaviorally oriented practitioner prefers to improve patient performance (let alone control status) by means other than compensatory lenses. Compensatory lenses should be considered only if they are constructive to the patient's performance and if the same degree of performance or better could not be achieved by a means designed to alter patient behavior. Probe tests of performance utilizing lateral yoked prisms and the Wirt Polaroid stereo test, as described in earlier chapters, have proven to be significant.

Similar use of yoked prisms on other stereo tests such as the Keystone Telebinocular DB6 (stereopsis) card is likewise significant. Recall that it is likely that lateral yoked prisms may alter the response on the Wirt test. One set (e.g., bases-right) could improve performance and the opposite base could reduce performance. If either or both is the case, this could indicate that the appropriate lateral yoked prisms should be incorporated in an appropriate total prescription temporarily. If this is the case, recall that the guideline for therapeutic purposes is to use the prism base that reduces the performance.

On the other hand, if the visual behavior is non-embedded and the stresspoint retinoscopy reveals the availability of equal plus spheres, the influence of such lenses on the Wirt test should be investigated and compared to the same probing with lateral yoked prisms. The following represent guidelines to prescribe:

1. If the counter-stress plus lenses improve the Wirt performance, no matter what influence lateral yoked prisms have, prescribe plus lenses only, preferably in Plano bifocals, assuming the condition requires no compensatory use of lenses.
2. If the counter-stress plus lenses do not alter the Wirt test results, but lateral yoked prisms do, prescribe the indicated lateral yoked prisms in bifocal form with the indicated counter-stress plus at near for constant wear for temporary therapeutic purposes.

Bear in mind that any lateral yoked prisms are deleted from the prescription when they no longer influence performance.

The more embedded the visual behavior, the more consideration must be given to the refractive status relative to lens prescription. Whether the patient's need is for near lenses or distant lenses, only that amount of difference is prescribed which is constructive to the patient's performance and needs.

Vertical imbalance is another less common manifestation of postural alteration—more often than not involving upper back and neck musculature (i.e., localization). The patient having vertical imbalance not related to trauma or paresis of extraocular musculature will generally reflect this postural adaptation on the way he carries his head and shoulders. Generally, he will only manifest this vertical deviancy to the optometrist when he is behind a phoropter, sitting in a position other than that which is peculiar and natural to him. He may manifest it to himself with recognition of diplopia if he deliberately alters or is forced to alter his body torque.

In the consideration of prescribing compensatory vertical prisms, it has long been recognized that if prism compensation is provided to this type of individual, he may accept it and even like it. When he returns to the optometrist, he might even reveal an increased vertical imbalance.

Actually, his mode of adaptation has been interfered with under these conditions. He needs, in turn, to alter himself further. Therefore, the general rule is to avoid prescribing compensatory vertical prisms unless diplopia is manifest without it. If the latter is the case, minimum vertical prism, usually evenly distributed between the two lenses, is prescribed to alleviate the diplopia.

CHAPTER 12
The Final Chapter:
Only a Beginning

This is the last chapter of "Lens Power in Action." However, it is not the final chapter of the topic.

It is virtually impossible to write a final chapter. These chapters have covered a great many areas, and have attempted to provide insight, by example, to the use of lenses from the behavioral concept of vision. This book has not covered all areas, and those that have been covered still leave some questions. Undoubtedly, additional questions have been created. In addition to anything else remaining to be explored related to the alteration of behavior and the power of lenses, three topics which stand out strongly in this author's mind are as follows: presbyopia, developmental guidance, and the use of lenses in visual training. Perhaps, in the near future, this author will once again take up the challenge and attempt to elaborate on these subjects. Hopefully, others will do likewise.

Writing has many rewards. The greatest reward to this author has been to receive questions triggered in readers' minds by these chapters. Many questions have been received during the course of these volumes. In turn, the questions have been answered directly.

This chapter will share some of these questions and answers. It has been particularly pleasing to note that many (not all) of the questions relate to the Skeffington Analytical Sequence (SAS) examination, its importance, and the insight derived by virtue of its use. The following questions were asked about the analytical examination:

1. How important is it to do a complete analytical examination?
2. Is the SAS analytical examination sequence critical to the behavioral concept?
3. Is the philosophy of the SAS synonymous with the behavioral approach to optometry?
4. Is the philosophy of lens fitting derived from the SAS equivalent to the behavioral concept of vision?
5. How important is it to do the analytical examination exactly as directed—both in sequence as well as methods?
6. Is the SAS analytical examination sequence, as taught by the late A. M. Skeffington, O.D., really necessary, unique, needed and viable?

7. Why take the time to do the analytical examination when any decision for lens values is derived from stresspoint retinoscopy and specific performance tests with yoked prisms?
8. Why do you do only partial analytical examinations on progress case studies?
9. Why do you use Plano as the control for many of the analytical findings when the #7 (subjective) is in plus? Isn't this contrary to the basic instructions?
10. Have you ever seen a perfect analytical, but the patient has a visual problem?

These are 10 very important and thought-provoking questions, many of which this author has taken for granted over the years because of his involvement and activity. It was not until these questions emerged that it was realized that these issues must be addressed and that possibly, for as long as a generation, many of us have been at fault by assuming that everyone was aware of the answers to these questions.

According to this author, the analytical examination, its sequence, and its methodology is to optometry what apple pie is to America. Historically, Dr. A. M. Skeffington created the analytical examination sequence with the contributions and support of his colleagues and associates. Initially, it was a "15-point" examination, then an "18-point" examination, and ultimately, with further elaboration, the more commonly known "21-point" examination sequence. The purpose of this examination sequence was to provide the clinician of the day with a means to determine a lens formula derived from the interpretation of the data collected that a patient could wear comfortably and satisfy his identified needs of the day. The method was born of the need created in the early days of formal optometric education when optometric students were taught "Ivory Castle" concepts of vision and lens prescribing, which patients rejected. This contrasted with the success in lens fitting enjoyed by those clinicians who had either no formal optometric education or minimal education.

Dr. Skeffington derived insight and information as to what and how they practiced and drew conclusions, discovered commonalities, and, ultimately, put it together in a sequence with guidelines that could be taught. History reveals that a profession was truly created as a product of this method. Insofar as the fundamental purpose of the method is concerned, there is no better, no faster and no more reliable means to examine vision and prescribe a safe and wearable lens formula.

"...the Skeffington Analytical Sequence is neither philosophy- nor concept-bound."

When E. B. Alexander, O.D., founded the Optometric Extension Program, Dr. Skeffington brought the then-developed analytical examination sequence and directive of lens application to the OEP. It is most important to bear in mind that the SAS method is neither philosophy- nor concept-bound, and it supercedes any theoretical base. In other words, the examination/analysis method does not represent any theory of vision or vision, itself. It is simply the SAS method, not an OEP philosophy.

However, this does not mean that some vision concept did not have some influence at the time in the consideration of specific tests and understanding that emerged with the method. After all, in the late 1920's, through the 1930's and into the 1940's, the existing vision concepts were either "optical" or "accommodative-convergence," and, in reality, the concept inherent in the accommodative-convergence notion influenced some aspects of the formulation of the analytical examination sequence and method.

Relative to current optometric education, the method should be taught and it can be taught easily in any existing college of optometry no matter what underlying vision concept prevails. The method, itself, does not imply a particular concept of vision. In fact, if such were the case, it would be a blessing because the present status in most colleges, insofar as examination and prescribing are concerned, suggests the "days of old" in the vision care field—applying what is known as "flying by the seat of their pants" and/or the old adage of "seven and four and out the door." Students are frustrated, and this has contributed to the search for a broader field outside optometry (e.g., the medical model) because their view of basic vision care is so small and limited. However, every college teaches the students how to do all of the tests of the analytical examination — although frequently not with all the controls and in the sequence dictated by the SAS method. The students just do not know the importance of and how to derive benefit from the test data. Thus, they put it to no use and, ultimately, do not even do the tests.

This author has long emphasized that it is inappropriate to speak of an OEP philosophy or concept. There is no such thing as an OEP philosophy of vision. On the other hand, it is proper to speak of the SAS method of case analysis and lens prescribing which is, in itself, solely the analytical examination sequence and subsequent analysis of the data collected by means of checking, chaining and typing the data, and subjecting the data to the seven directives of lens application from which is derived the safe, wearable lens formula.

The OEP is an educational institution committed to continuous continuing optometric education, not a concept of vision. As an institution, it has had its bias in the past, as well as in the present. Hopefully, it always will. It has provided the opportunity for the late Dr. Skeffington and others to develop what today we refer to as the behavioral concept of vision. It provides the platform for the behavioral aspects of optometry, but OEP IS NOT behavioral optometry. Equating the two is both inappropriate and detrimental both to OEP and optometry. On the other hand, OEP's present dedication to the teaching of the behavioral concept is most important.

Likewise, it is just as inappropriate to equate OEP with visual training, the behavioral aspects of optometry with visual training, OEP with children's vision, visual training with children, and so on. The behavioral concept is not a specific treatment program or optometric program of care. It is a concept of vision from which guidelines for optometric care emerge, which can result in the prescription of lenses or in formalized visual training.

"The Skeffington Analytical Sequence is one thing and the behavioral concept is another."

Again (at the risk of being overly redundant, yet deliberately so), it is important to emphasize that the SAS method is one thing and the behavioral concept is another. This perspective always must be remembered. This leads to the all-important questions of (1) "Why does an optometrist with a behavioral orientation to vision care do the SAS analytical examination sequence?" and (2) "Why does the an optometrist providing a behavioral approach to vision care do the SAS case analysis?"

Assuming patient capability, this author does the complete analytical examination sequence with every new patient and with every regular patient of the practice seen for his or her annual programmed optometric reevaluation examination. The analytical examination sequence is one of a number of tests and investigations conducted in the course of a complete examination. As one test, it is comprised of a series of probes (analytical sequence numbers 3 through 21) and it requires about 12 minutes to complete. Particularly for the data to be significant both to the SAS method and to the behavioral concept, the probes, with rare exception, must be done specifically as taught by the "black book", using the stated sequence, the stated condition, and the instructional sets. Any deviations can reduce the validity and reliability of the data derived from these probes when used to determine the safe, wearable lens formula as well as understand and derive conclusions for a given patient from the behavioral viewpoint.

Thus, one reason to do the analytical examination sequence is that it provides the necessary data from which can be determined, in the most reliable means, the safe lens prescribable—representing both the conventional approach to vision care and this author's number one alternative of optometric care. This, of course, represents minimum level vision care and this author feels obligated to offer this level as one alternative to his patients.

> ***"...the analytical examination sequence...is essential to provide appropriate optometric care vis-à-vis the behavioral concept of vision."***

The most important reason to do the analytical examination sequence in the current era is that data derived from this test is essential to provide appropriate optometric care vis-à-vis the behavioral concept of vision. This author knows of no other way to do the same. (Perhaps there are other means and methods of investigation to derive the same insight. No one has shown or demonstrated this to the author yet.) The data of the analytical examination, in conjunction with other performance data gathered in the course of the optometric examination, is essential for the optometrist to understand and to guide his patient. Specific to any consideration of the behavioral concept, it is essential that we know the status of adaptation in time, let alone the nature of the adaptation if adverse. Therefore, the data of the analytical examination is essential to know the degree of embeddedness. Presently, this author knows no other way than analysis of this data to learn this status. This information is essential to know the predicted value of a program of optometric care and benefits to be derived for any given patient.

Recall that the behavioral concept suggests that lenses can be utilized to prevent, protect, control, maintain, and enhance. Nowhere in the analytical examination sequence is such a lens formula to be found. Such a lens formula is not one that has been determined by the utilization of the seven directives of lens application. Such a lens is not equivalent to the #14 (cross cylinder) nets as has been erroneously suggested and taught in some colleges of optometry. This author has expressed his opinion in past chapters of these volumes that the most direct means to determine the counter-stress lens formula is the stresspoint retinoscopic procedure and, secondly, bell retinoscopy. Other than the clinician's professional judgment, feeling tone, and "flying by the seat of the pants" (and just guessing), this author knows of no other way.

On the other hand, the value and essence of the analytical examination sequence data is that the optometrist, by virtue of knowing the status of embeddedness, can predict the benefits to the patient by utilizing such lenses. In other words, the analytical examination data does not provide the behavioral concept lens formula. However, appropriate interpretation of the data gives insight insofar as value to the patient is concerned. This is significant to the optometrist from another angle, in that it influences the fee. Recall that the patient, in the final analysis, pays for benefits to be derived from the optometric care program—the greater the benefits predicted, the higher the fee.

The question was raised relative to the analytical examination sequence and progress case studies. It was noted that in reporting patient data during office visits subsequent to the original complete diagnostic examination, only part of the complete analytical sequence data was reported or recorded. Is this true? If so, why? When the patient returns for progress case studies, that is, reevaluation examinations other than the complete annual examination, the patient is exposed only to those probes of the analytical sequence (in addition to other tests) which are essential to this author's understanding of his or her movement in time. This author gathers data essential for comparison and data related to benefits derived as well as additional benefits and expectations that can be predicted.

Inherent in the structure of the instructions to perform the analytical examination sequence is the directive related to the lens control through which the patient views when doing probes beyond the #7 (subjective). The basic rules are as follows:

1. Distance findings (#10 [base-out break/recovery] and #11 [base-in break/recover]) are taken with #7 (subjective) in place.
2. Near findings (#16 [base-out break/recovery], #17 [base-in break/recovery], #20 [positive relative accommodation], #21 [negative relative accommodation]) are taken with #7 (subjective) in place, if the patient is capable of resolving 20/20 type at near; if not, use and record as the control lenses that which permits him or her to do so. As the behavioral concept evolved and we viewed the data of the probes from another point of view, the suggestion arose that the data possibly would be even more meaningful if, in the case of an individual with unaided visual acuity of 20/20 (and with no prior habitual constant wear prescription) the probes were performed through Plano (the habitual condition). Basic to the analytical method, the base-out and base-in to break measurements were critical to determine case typing.

The question evolving was whether the control lens formula would influence these findings and alter case typing. If it did, perhaps it would be best to maintain the basic guidelines. On the other hand, if it did not alter the case typing, there might be more insight to be gained by taking these findings through the habitual status. Indeed, subsequent personal comparative investigation on the part of the author revealed that the quantitative values of these probes in question could vary depending on the formula used as control (for example, #7 (subjective) or Plano), but the case typing did not alter. The implication was that the application of the directives of lens application would not be modified if the control formula was altered. Yet, the insight to be gained related to investigation of performance under habitual conditions could be increased. Thus, for many years, this author used Plano as control for distance findings and Plano for near findings, assuming one had unaided visual acuity of 20/20 and no habitual constant wear prescription. If the patient had worn a specific prescription for near, the near findings were taken through this. In the final analysis, there was nothing to lose by altering this one condition; yet, potentially, there was a lot of insight to be gained.

Finally, the question was raised as to whether this author has "ever seen a perfect analytical but the patient has a visual problem?" This question, in turn, leads to additional questions because there are some underlying implications inherent in the question itself. For example, what is meant by a perfect analytical? What is meant by a visual problem? It is conceivable that what is meant by a perfect analytical is a resulting analytical examination sequence in which the data of the individual probes either matched or exceeded the analytical expecteds. If this is the case, the underlying implication is that the expecteds are equivalent to that expected idealistically of the unimpaired individual.

Nothing could be further from the truth, relative to the purpose and utilization of the expecteds. The expecteds are not to be considered anything more than what was intended. They do not represent the unimpaired. Nor do they represent the norm or normal visual performance.

Referring once again to past history, the expecteds were established as a product of experience and insight drawn from the experiences of Dr. Skeffington, his colleagues and associates. They represented a base line from which comparisons could be drawn for the purpose of checking, chaining, and typing the collected data, purely and simply.

Interestingly enough, at least three studies were done years ago, two of which were designed ultimately to deny the teaching of Skeffington and the SAS by investigating the findings of the analytical sequence. As it turned out, all three studies substantiated the expecteds as being reliable figures. From this was derived an inappropriate conclusion that these expecteds were norms.

"The analytical findings do not reveal a disability, but they can infer a disability."

Further appraisal of the expecteds, as if they represented a given individual, would reveal that they conform to the expected behavior associated with embeddedness. Here again, this was not the purpose and should not be interpreted as such. The analytical findings do not reveal a disability, but they can infer a disability. The analytical examination, as emphasized earlier, is but one test. On the other hand, as Tole Greenstein, O.D., so frequently stated relative to a visual problem, "If it's in the person, it's in the analytical." Thus, 'tis but a matter of data evaluation and interpretation.

If the use of the term *visual problem* is in reference to an identifiable disability in the visual process, it could be assumed that it would be highly unlikely that the analytical examination data would match the expecteds. This is not because the expecteds are the ideal, but, rather, because that which represents the probes would be affected in various ways and reflected in the findings. If, on the other hand, the term visual problem is used as defined in these chapters ("a visually-oriented unsatisfied personal need"), it is conceivable that a visual problem could exist and the analytical examination sequence findings can be equivalent to or exceed the expecteds. However, the author does not necessarily recall such an individual—not due to an inadequate memory, but to the fact that he does not view the analytical data in the light of the question's implication.

As these chapters draw to a close, I want to express my sincere appreciation to the Optometric Extension Program Foundation for affording me the opportunity to express in this format how we view and apply the underlying principles of the behavioral concept of vision. I also want to express my appreciation to all the readers of these chapters for the opportunity to share and communicate and especially for the opportunity to carry on additional communication by answering the questions raised by the chapters. Hopefully, every answer has led to at least one or more additional questions.

Certainly, additional questions remain to be answered. There is no end, no conclusion, and hopefully, there never will be. After all, let us trust that there will be no end to growth and development in ourselves, our thinking, and the clinical expertise to which we dedicate ourselves.

The discipline of vision (optometry) and the profession of vision care (optometry) are broader than how we perceive them today. There is no question that the visual process is dominant. Yet, even to this day, the very extent and implication of this statement is not totally known. It is my hope and personal intention, that all of us will continue to explore this unknown—and gradually learn more, know more, and do more for people and their vision.

VISION - the deriving of meaning and the directing of action as a product of processing information triggered by a selected band of radiant energy.